Comments on *Chronic Obstructive Pulmonary Disease in Primary Care* from readers

It provides a wealth of practical information for all health professionals who work in general practice.

Greta Barnes, Founder of the
National Respiratory Training Centre

This is an exceptional piece of work and one that I hope will be taken extremely seriously within Primary Health Care.

Lynn Young, Royal College of Nursing

I think that this is an extremely clearly written book, which is clearly going to be extremely important in highlighting the role of primary care in managing patients with COPD. It is amazing that such a comprehensive book on COPD in primary care had not previously been written, and I think that this publication fills that hole extremely well!

Michael Rudolf, Consultant Physician,
Ealing Hospital

COPD in Primary Care *really is excellent. I particularly like the logical layout of the text, making it easy to dip in and out and pick up the bits one is interested in.*

E Neville, Consultant Physician
St Mary's Hospital, Portsmouth

This is required reading for anyone involved in the multi-disciplinary approach to COPD Management. It is clear, concise and above all gives a common sense approach to this difficult but important problem.

Dr R N Harrison, Consultant Physician,
Respiratory Unit, North Tees and Hartlepool NHS Trust

It is without doubt the best book available for general practitioners who want a comprehensive account in chronic obstructive pulmonary disease.

Professor J J Reid, Head of the Department of General Practice,
University of Otago, New Zealand

Reviews of *Chronic Obstructive Pulmonary Disease in Primary Care*

This is a much needed, very practical book, clearly laid out with a main points section at the start of each chapter and references at the end of the chapter. A useful addition to the practice bookshelf.

Practical Nursing

COPD in Primary Care *fills in the gaps in advising on day-to-day management following the launch of the British Thoracic Guidelines for COPD, and shows that COPD is an important condition that can effectively be dealt with in primary care. If you want to know how ... this book is for you!*

National Respiratory Training Centre

This book continues to represent excellent value and a good starting point for any doctor or nurse interested in learning more about the essentials of managing COPD.

Extract from a review on COPD Professional.org website

This book, which has been endorsed by the Australian Lung Foundation and the Thoracic Society of Australia and New Zealand, is a goldmine of practical information on the management of a condition that is increasing in incidence and prevalence in our community. I thoroughly recommend it to all medical practitioners who manage chronic lung disease, especially those who are engaged in comprehensive care from the consultation room, through the hospital ward, to the community setting.

Medicine Today
about the Australian edition

Chronic Obstructive Pulmonary Disease in Primary Care

Third edition

All you need to know to manage COPD in your practice

Dr David Bellamy MBE, BSc, FRCP, MRCGP, DRCOG

GP Principal with a special interest in respiratory medicine at the James Fisher Medical Centre, Bournemouth
Member of the COPD Guidelines Committee

and

Rachel Booker RGN DN(Cert)HV

COPD module leader for the National Respiratory Training Centre, Warwick
Member of the British Thoracic Society COPD Consortium

Class Publishing • London

Text © David Bellamy and Rachel Booker 2000, 2002, 2004
© Class Publishing 2000, 2002, 2004

The information presented in this book is accurate and current to the best of the authors' knowledge. The authors and publisher, however, make no guarantee as to, and assume no responsibility for, the correctness, sufficiency or completeness of such information or recommendation.

Printing history
First published 2000
Reprinted 2000
Second edition 2002
Reprinted 2003
Third edition 2004

The authors and publisher welcome feedback from the users of this book. Please contact the publisher:

Class Publishing (London) Ltd,
Barb House, Barb Mews,
London W6 7PA
Telephone: 020 7371 2119
Fax 020 7371 2878 [International +4420]
Email: post@class.co.uk
Website: www.class.co.uk

A CIP catalogue record for this book is available from the British Library

ISBN 1 85959 104 3

Edited by Gillian Clarke

Designed and typeset by Martin Bristow

Indexed by Valerie Elliston

Line illustrations by David Woodroffe

Printed and bound in Slovenia by Delo Tiskarna
by arrangement with Prešernova družba

Contents

Foreword

by Dr David Halpin DPhil, FRCP
*Consultant Physician and Senior Lecturer in Respiratory
Medicine, Royal Devon & Exeter Hospital
Chairman of the NICE COPD Guideline Committee*

The fact that this is the third edition of *Chronic Obstructive Pulmonary Disease* reflects two important points. Firstly, it is a tribute to the success of the first two editions in which the authors have used their considerable experience to provide clear information and practical advice about the management of COPD. Secondly, it reflects the accelerating pace of progress in COPD management that has occurred in the last few years. COPD is now firmly on the primary care agenda. In the UK, this is partly as a result of the new General Practice contract but also because of the publication of the NICE guidelines on the management of COPD and the introduction of new and more effective therapies. There is no longer any excuse for those commissioning health services to ignore COPD, and this book will help primary care clinicians develop services for people with COPD and implement the recommendations contained in the guidelines.

This edition contains a new chapter on the NICE guidelines and updated information on the GOLD guidelines in the light of the 2003 revision. It also discusses the role of the newer therapies.

There is much more interest in the management of COPD in primary care than there was when the first edition was published. We all face the challenge of providing multidisciplinary care for patients with this multi-component disease and I have no doubt that the latest edition of this book will greatly assist in this process.

Foreword to the first edition

by Greta Barnes MBE
Founder of the National Respiratory Training Centre

In recent years alterations in health care and health policy have accelerated change in the management of chronic diseases such as diabetes, asthma and hypertension. There has been an increasing shift of emphasis from secondary to primary care, and a collaborative approach has been encouraged not only between hospital and general practice but also between GP and practice nurse.

By 2020 chronic obstructive pulmonary disease (COPD), the 'smokers' disease', is likely to become the UK's fifth most common cause of death. It will also be managed chiefly in the community. At present it has been acknowledged that COPD is not widely understood by the vast majority of doctors and nurses, particularly in primary care. Many patients may have been misdiagnosed and therefore inappropriately treated.

The publication of *Chronic Obstructive Pulmonary Disease in Primary Care* has proved very timely. It gives a wealth of practical information for all health professionals who work in general practice. The authors highlight the importance of correct diagnosis and the value of spirometry as well as how to treat and manage the patient with COPD. The chapter on smoking cessation, which is the single most important intervention, provides invaluable advice to the reader, as does the section on ways to improve the quality of life for patients with this debilitating condition.

David Bellamy and Rachel Booker have a wealth of experience looking after COPD patients in general practice. In this book they have demonstrated the value of combining medical and nursing experience so that they can help others strive for excellence.

Undoubtedly this book will attract a wide range of health professionals who work in the community. It will also serve admirably to complement the National Respiratory Training Centre's Chronic Obstructive Pulmonary Disease Training Programme.

The authors are to be congratulated on producing a much-needed book – the first of its kind for primary care.

Foreword to the first edition

by Professor Peter Calverley MB, FRCP, FRCPE
Professor of Medicine (Pulmonary and Rehabilitation),
The University of Liverpool

Chronic obstructive pulmonary disease is a common, often unrecognised, source of morbidity and mortality in the UK and throughout the world. Traditionally, it has been seen as a 'dull' condition devoid of exciting symptoms or physical signs that help enliven the teaching of medical students and largely unresponsive to treatment. This therapeutic failure on the doctor's part is often excused by the recognition that the condition itself is usually brought on by cigarette smoking and therefore is 'the patient's own fault'. This has led to a type of therapeutic nihilism, which can no longer be justified given the changes in our understanding of the causes and consequences of COPD as well as the availability of more effective treatments. Despite encouraging reductions in the use of cigarettes, especially by middle-aged men, the problems of the COPD patient persist and are likely to do so even in the developed economies of the world. Patients who might have succumbed from their illness had they continued smoking in the past now develop symptoms related to their previous lung damage as they age, and this respiratory disability is an increasing burden to all those involved in the care of older patients. We now have the techniques relatively readily available to help make a firm diagnosis of COPD and to distinguish these patients from the many others with a bewildering array of similar symptoms produced by different pathologies, where the therapeutic approach and the likely prognosis will vary. The management of the COPD patient is increasingly multidisciplinary and the patients themselves are entitled to explanations not only of how their disease arises but also what the different treatments recommended do and what kind of improvement they are likely to achieve. The dilemma for health professionals is that this type of information has often not been available to them during their training, nor is it sufficiently up to date to help them form a useful management plan. This book has set out to remedy these problems.

This short book provides a wealth of information and practical advice, based on clinical experience and evidence-based recommendations. It is written by a general practitioner and a nurse educator, both with wide experience of respiratory disease and who are familiar with the kinds of questions that someone new to this field is bound to ask. They stress the importance of a positive diagnosis and of a positive therapeutic approach. When the correct patients are identified, useful things can be done for them even if this is unlikely to completely abolish all their symptoms once the disease itself is advanced.

The authors have been keen to demystify the role of pulmonary function testing while indicating how it fits into everyday clinical management. Their recommendations are up to date, and include some of the very latest clinical trial data as well as practical comments about the management of complications and acute exacerbations of disease. The result is a handbook of practical information that will be helpful to everyone concerned with this common clinical problem.

Hopefully, those who read and use this book will feel more confident about managing COPD in their daily practice, which in turn will begin to reverse the expectations of patients and doctors that, in the past, have been so low but no longer need to be quite so pessimistic.

Acknowledgements

We thank Greta Barnes, Founder of the National Respiratory Training Centre, and Richard Harrison, consultant respiratory physician at Stockton on Tees. Without their encouragement, this book would never have been started.

We also thank both our families for their support and tolerance.

Abbreviations

AHR airway hyper-responsiveness

AMP adenosine monophosphate

BMI body mass index

BTS British Thoracic Society

CT computed tomography

FEV$_1$ forced expired volume produced in the first second

FEV$_1$/FVC% the ratio of FEV$_1$ to FVC, expressed as a percentage

FVC forced vital capacity – the total volume of air that can be exhaled from maximal inhalation to maximal exhalation

IL interleukin

JVP jugular venous pressure

LRTI lower respiratory tract infection

LTOT long-term oxygen treatment

MDI metered dose inhaler

NE neutrophil elastase

NOTT Nocturnal Oxygen Therapy Trial

NRT nicotine replacement therapy

NSAID non-steroidal anti-inflammatory drug

OSA obstructive sleep apnoea

Paco_2 arterial carbon dioxide tension

Pao_2 arterial oxygen tension

PDE phosphodiesterase

PEF peak expiratory flow – the maximal flow rate that can be maintained over the first 10 milliseconds of a forced blow

RV residual (lung) volume

TLC total lung capacity

TLco diffusing capacity for carbon monoxide, or diffusing capacity

TNF tumour necrosis factor

VC (relaxed or slow) vital capacity

1 | Introduction

Main points

1   COPD is a common and important respiratory disorder that causes considerable morbidity and patient suffering.

2   It comprises a spectrum of diseases, including chronic bronchitis, emphysema, long-standing asthma that is no longer reversible and small airways disease.

3   COPD is a chronic, slowly progressive disorder characterised by airflow obstruction that varies very little from month to month.

4   The main cause of COPD is cigarette smoking.

5   COPD is more common in men and with increasing age. The prevalence is 2% of men aged 45–65 and 7% of men over 75 years. Some 32,000 people die from COPD each year in the UK.

6   It results in a large economic burden to the nation in excess of £800 million per year for health care.

7   The symptoms of breathlessness and coughing increasingly affect levels of activity, work, lifestyle and social interaction.

8   The first set of British clinical guidelines was published by the British Thoracic Society in 1997. Much new therapy and clinical information has appeared since then, and new evidence-based guidelines have thus been compiled by the National Institute for Clinical Excellence (NICE) and were published in February 2004 to update knowledge and best management. The new material comprises Chapter 11.

9   Other guidelines around the world are also being updated, including a new version of the global guidelines, GOLD, produced jointly by the National Heart, Lung and Blood Institute (NHLBI) and the World Health Organization (WHO).

What is new in this third edition

The main aim of producing this new edition is to add all the important evidence-based knowledge and changes in treatment that have been reviewed by NICE and published in new guidelines in February 2004. These guidelines, produced in conjunction with the British Thoracic Society and representatives of primary care, are likely to form the basis of good COPD clinical care for the next four to five years. A new chapter (Chapter 11) outlines the important new changes and main themes of continuing, relevant, management.

The GOLD Guidelines were updated in 2003 and this edition contains the new management changes.

The NICE Guidelines emphasise the central role of the patient and the need to involve patients much more in management and decision making. Good COPD management requires a multidisciplinary approach, not only from doctors and nurses in primary and secondary care but also from physiotherapists, dietitians, pharmacists, occupational therapists, counsellors and social services.

The timing of a new edition is very opportune because, in the UK, a new Primary Care GP contract came into force in April 2004 and COPD is one of the disease areas for better care and audit. Furthermore, the Primary Care Collaborative, a body sponsored by the Department of Health, has selected COPD and diabetes for improving the standards of management and data collection.

The combination of these three initiatives should raise the profile of COPD and provide the much-needed impetus to better diagnosis and management of this common and disabling disease.

Why COPD is important

Chronic obstructive pulmonary disease (COPD) is one of the most common and important respiratory disorders in primary care. About 32,000 people die from COPD each year in the UK, and the disease results in considerable morbidity, impaired quality of life, time off work, and more hospital admissions and GP consultations than asthma. However, its diagnosis and effective management have been largely neglected, apart from patients being advised to stop smoking.

COPD is a spectrum of diseases that includes:

- chronic bronchitis,

- emphysema,

- long-standing asthma that has become relatively unresponsive to treatment,

- small airways disease.

The unifying feature of COPD is that it is a chronic, slowly progressive disorder characterised by airflow obstruction that is not fully reversible and varies very little from day to day and month to month.

COPD is caused mainly by cigarette smoking. However, only 20% of smokers will develop COPD and there are no clear pointers to what makes them particularly susceptible to the adverse effects of tobacco smoke. It is probable that there are genetic factors that increase susceptibility to smoking but, as yet, no chromosomal abnormalities have been identified other than for alpha-1 antitrypsin deficiency. Family studies have found that siblings of people with emphysema are three to four times more likely than controls to develop COPD if they smoke. For people who are affected, stopping smoking is the only way to slow the progression of the disease. There are as yet no drugs that significantly improve the disease or alter the rate of decline of lung function.

The 1990s saw great improvements in the management and organisation of asthma treatment in primary care. COPD, by contrast, has been largely ignored and rightly has been dubbed the 'Cinderella respiratory disorder'. This situation began to change with the publication and widespread dissemination to GPs and practice nurses of the British Thoracic Society (BTS) *COPD Guidelines* in December 1997. Since then there has been considerable interest in the disease and its management. Research papers on COPD have flourished at both British and international meetings. The BTS Guidelines have set out five goals for COPD management:

- early and accurate diagnosis,

- best control of symptoms,

- prevention of deterioration,

- prevention of complications,

- improved quality of life.

Guidelines are important in aiding accurate and appropriate clinical decision-making but are not useful unless disseminated to all primary care doctors and practice nurses in a simple, readily digestible format. The BTS COPD Consortium produced a four-page summary of the 1997 Guidelines, which was widely distributed to primary care. The Consortium will similarly distribute a short summary of the NICE guidelines shortly after publication, with more detailed information available to view and download from the BTS website. The full guideline appeared as a supplement of *Thorax* in March 2004.

How important is COPD?

The most up-to-date figures suggest that 1.5% of the UK population have been diagnosed with COPD – a total of 900,000 people. Men are more likely to be affected than women, with prevalence rates of 2% in men aged 45–65 years and 7% in men over 75. The rates for women are rising, however, which is probably related to their increased smoking over the last 20 years. These figures are likely to be an under-estimate of the true prevalence, because much COPD may be mis-labelled as asthma. Moreover, most mild COPD goes unrecognised because patients are relatively asymptomatic, with only minor symptoms such as a smoker's cough or mild breathlessness on exertion. As a result, they often don't consult their doctor. Recent studies indicate that as few as 1 person in 4 with COPD is recognised.

In 1999, COPD accounted for 7.4% of all deaths among men and 4.1% among women in the UK. Mortality tends to be greater in urban areas, particularly in South Wales, the north-west of England and Scotland. There is a strong association with lower social class and poverty that can be explained only partly by the higher smoking rates of this group.

On a more global basis, the WHO estimates the prevalence of COPD to be 600 million world-wide. COPD is currently the fifth greatest cause of mortality world-wide, with over 2.5 million deaths recorded in 2000. By 2020, COPD is projected to become the third leading cause of death and the fifth leading cause of morbidity. Most other chronic diseases, including coronary artery disease, strokes and cancer, are likely to decrease over this period.

A project for the future – when suitable government funding is made available – might be to screen smokers over the age of 45 years with spirometry (see Chapter 4) to detect early airflow obstruction before symptoms start. It will still be difficult to persuade people at risk to stop smoking but, if they are successful at this point of the disease, most of them will never develop symptomatic COPD. This will produce major personal benefits for them as well as a significant cost saving to the NHS.

As the disease progresses, patients become increasingly short of breath – washing, getting dressed and minimal exertion become difficult. The effect on lifestyle can be devastating, resulting in physical suffering, mood change and depression, together with social isolation. Many sufferers will have to accept early retirement, which can create financial problems for them. Even at a less severe level, many activities are restricted:

- doing jobs around the house,
- hobbies (e.g. gardening),
- choice of holiday venues.

When one partner is significantly restricted, a marriage may be put under considerable strain.

An important part of COPD management is to be aware of these problems. Addressing social and psychological needs as well as encouraging patients to take as much regular exercise as possible should form an integral part of their care. Information on disability grants and aids, such as the Blue (formerly Orange) Badge parking scheme for people with disabilities, may help improve their overall quality of life.

What is the economic burden of COPD?

The total cost of COPD to the UK health care system in 1996 was estimated at £817 million. Secondary care management accounts for over half the total and in 2001 amounted to £587 million for the UK. Over the last decade, admissions to hospital have increased by 50%.

In an average health district serving 250,000 people there will be 14,500 GP consultations every year. The average cost per patient per annum is £810.42, at least three times the cost of a patient with asthma. Of this figure, 54.3% is due to in-patient care, 18.6% for treatment, 16.4% for GP contact, 5.7% for A & E visits and 5% for tests. Not surprisingly, the cost per patient dramatically increases with disease severity from £150 per year with mild disease, to £308 with moderate disease and £1,307 with severe disease.

A typical COPD patient consults 2.4 times per year, and has an estimated mean annual drug bill of £124. Oxygen therapy is an expensive part of treatment and the data suggest that oxygen is not being used most economically. About 30,000 patients with COPD receive oxygen therapy, and 23,000 of them use oxygen cylinders. The annual cost of regular use of oxygen by cylinder is £6,500 per patient, whereas the running costs of an oxygen concentrator are only £900 per year.

Patients with severe COPD often experience exacerbations of their symptoms – which are a common reason for their being admitted to hospital. A survey in Merseyside calculated that 12.5% of all medical acute admissions were for exacerbations of COPD. In an average health district the annual inpatient bed days amount to 9,600, compared with 1,800 for asthma. The length of stay is notably longer than for asthma: 10 days for COPD compared with 3.6 days for asthma.

COPD also causes considerable loss of time from work – 24 million days in 1994/5. The economic cost for that period amounted to £600 million in state benefits. Adding the value of lost work to employers brings the total economic cost to the nation to a staggering £2.7 billion!

Doctors' and patients' attitudes to COPD

The medical profession in both primary and secondary care has traditionally had a negative view of COPD, despite how often patients consult about it. Some of the reasons include:

- it is an illness for which little can be done,
- it is regarded as a self-inflicted illness,
- there is generally a low level of interest among primary care doctors,
- it has a low profile in the NHS,
- there is little incentive and time to set up early screening,
- inadequate use of spirometry,

■ poor understanding of spirometric technique and interpretation of results,

■ inadequate access to hospital testing of respiratory function,

■ missed opportunities when seeing COPD patients (or potential early COPD patients) during acute respiratory infections.

The general public are not well informed, either, and, even when symptoms are present, people seem reluctant to see their GP about the condition. A survey conducted on behalf of the British Thoracic Society's COPD Consortium in 2001 interviewed 866 adults about their knowledge of COPD and its symptoms. Only 35% had heard of the term 'COPD' whereas 92% had heard of chronic bronchitis and 79% had heard of emphysema. Just under 30% of the sample had experienced breathlessness on mild exertion and 22% frequent winter coughs and colds. When symptomatic people were asked if they had visited a GP with these symptoms only 54% said yes. The reasons given by 65% of them were that they were either not bothered by the symptoms or were unaware they needed to be checked by a doctor. Another 23% said they would not go to the surgery, as the GP would just tell them to stop smoking. A further 21% were too busy.

The data from this survey highlight the considerable obstacles there are to finding and diagnosing the early stages of the disease.

Identifying patients

People with or at risk of COPD can be identified by the following measures.

■ Evaluating and optimising treatment in those with an existing diagnosis of chronic bronchitis, emphysema or COAD.

■ Reviewing patients over 40 labelled as having asthma or those taking bronchodilators who also smoke.

■ Performing spirometry on smokers with breathlessness, cough, sputum or wheeze. Recalling smokers with acute bronchitis, when they are well, to perform lung function testing.

■ Screening of asymptomatic smokers over 35 – there may be as many as 20% with airflow obstruction. A case-controlled study by van Schayck in the Netherlands found that in smokers aged over 35 years who also have a persistent cough, 27% had airflow obstruction on spirometry.

■ Encouraging patients to report to their GP surgery if they have symptoms – the British Thoracic Society and the British Lung Foundation have posters that can be displayed in surgeries and pharmacies.

What can be done?

GPs and practice nurses can considerably improve the symptoms and lifestyle of patients with this very common disease. By making a correct diagnosis as early in the disease process as possible, maximum influence can be brought to bear on the patient to stop smoking and thus prevent the development of severe and disabling symptoms.

Once the disease is manifest, patients should be given the opportunity to have optimal bronchodilator therapy – the most important treatment to improve breathlessness and exercise tolerance. They need to be encouraged to exercise fully and to modify lifestyle factors, such as being overweight. The adverse social and psychological effects of the disease need to be recognised, carefully assessed and, where possible, alleviated. Patients with more severe disease may need to be referred to hospital for assessment for long-term oxygen, bronchodilators via nebuliser or possible surgery.

In the past the approach to managing COPD has been too negative. Much can be done for these patients, and primary care is the main site for their diagnosis and treatment. This book aims to equip you, as a primary care professional, to achieve this. NICE has put the COPD patient at the centre of management and decision-making.

In 2003 the Respiratory Alliance, a group representing primary and secondary care, nurses and patient groups, produced a report on improving high-quality integrated respiratory care called *Bridging the Gap*. In it they set out the following 'reasonable expectations' for patients with COPD.

■ All smokers have the right to co-ordinated smoking cessation services.

■ They have the right to timely and accurate diagnosis.

- They have the right to management in line with approved guidelines.

- They have the right to access pulmonary rehabilitation services from an early stage in their disease.

- They have the right to access appropriate secondary care services.

- They have a right to appropriate assessment and practical support for the use of supplementary oxygen.

- They have a right to integrated health, social and palliative care services.

Further reading

Bridging the Gap – commissioning and delivering high quality integrated respiratory healthcare. A report from the Respiratory Alliance. 2003. Respiratory Alliance, Direct Publishing Solutions, Cookham, Berks

Burden of Lung Disease. A statistics report from the British Thoracic Society. November 2001. On the BTS website

Casting a shadow over the nation's health. Lung Report 111, 2003. On the British Lung Foundation website

VAN SCHAYCK CP, LOOZEN JM, WAGENA E et al. (2002) Detecting patients at high risk of developing chronic obstructive pulmonary disease in general practice; cross-sectional case-finding study. *British Medical Journal* **324**: 1370–4

Pathology and pathophysiology

Main points

1 COPD is not a discrete clinical entity, but a combination of emphysema, chronic bronchitis, small airways disease and chronic asthma.

2 The most important risk factor is cigarette smoking.

3 Treating persistent asthma early and aggressively with inhaled steroids may reduce the development of chronic airflow limitation.

4 Chronic mucus production alone is not always associated with the development of progressive airflow limitation; however, when there is progressive airflow limitation, chronic mucus production may accelerate the decline in lung function.

5 Emphysema is thought to develop as a result of an imbalance between elastase and anti-elastase activity in the lung.

6 Loss of lung elastin, such as occurs in emphysema, contributes to airway collapse, particularly during exercise.

7 Hyperinflation of the lungs leads to increased breathlessness on exertion.

8 Disruption of gas exchange leads to polycythaemia, cor pulmonale and respiratory failure.

COPD is not a single disease entity, but an overlapping syndrome of the four main conditions (Figure 2.1):

■ emphysema,

■ chronic bronchitis,

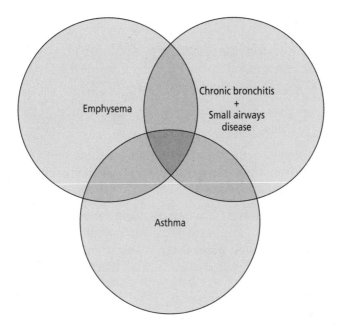

Figure 2.1 Diagrammatic representation of the four main conditions
that comprise COPD

■ small airways disease,

■ chronic asthma.

It has thus defied definition in terms of pathology. The National
Institute for Clinical Excellence (NICE) defines COPD as:

'characterised by airflow obstruction. The airflow obstruction
is usually progressive, not fully reversible and does not
change markedly over several months. The disease is
predominantly caused by smoking.'

GOLD guidelines similarly define COPD in functional terms but
both GOLD and NICE also allude to the underlying pathological
process and its cause. GOLD defines COPD as:

'a disease state characterised by airflow limitation that is not
fully reversible. The airflow limitation is both progressive and
associated with an abnormal inflammatory response of the
lungs to noxious particles or gases.'

NICE also states:

- Airflow obstruction is defined as a reduced FEV_1 ($FEV_1 < 80$ predicted) and a reduced FEV_1/FVC ratio (< 0.7). (FEV_1 and FVC are explained in Chapter 4.)

- The airflow obstruction is due to a combination of airway and parenchymal damage.

- The damage is the result of chronic inflammation which differs from that seen in asthma and which is usually the result of tobacco smoke.

Some patients have an asthmatic element to their COPD and it will be possible to reverse their airflow obstruction to some degree. However, even when there is an asthma element, the lung function *cannot be returned to normal*, no matter how intensive the treatment.

Risk factors

Cigarette smoking

Cigarette smoking is overwhelmingly the most important risk factor for the development of COPD. Indeed, this is reflected in the GOLD and NICE guidelines' definition of the disease. Although COPD can occur in non-smokers, about 90% of cases are thought to be a direct result of cigarette smoking.

Lung function declines after the age of 30–35 years as part of the ageing process (Figure 2.2).

- In normal, healthy non-smokers the rate of decline of FEV_1 is about 25–30ml a year.

- In 'at-risk' smokers the rate of decline may be double that, at about 50–60ml a year.

Why some smokers are at risk of this accelerated decline and others are not has been the subject of considerable research. Involvement of genetic factors is suggested by the 'clustering' of COPD cases in some families. Although some of this increased risk may be due to shared environmental factors, studies of diverse populations suggest that shared environment does not provide a full

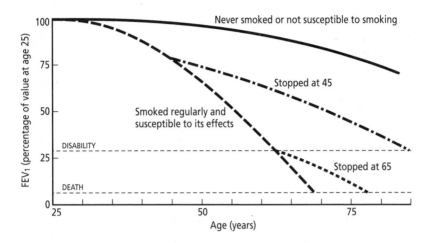

Figure 2.2 The decline in lung function as part of the normal ageing process and as accelerated by cigarette smoking.
(Reproduced, with permission, from Fletcher and Peto, 1977)

explanation. The search for a 'COPD gene' has revealed a number of possible candidates, but has so far been inconclusive.

What is known is that lung function declines steadily over the years of smoking but the FEV_1 often drops below 50% of predicted before symptoms appear. Patients usually present with symptoms of COPD between the ages of 50 and 70 years.

Although lost lung function is not regained when smoking is stopped, the rate of decline returns to that of a non-smoker or non-susceptible smoker (see Figure 2.2). This highlights the importance of the early detection of such high-risk smokers and persuading them to stop smoking. If they can be persuaded to stop, they may never suffer from severe, disabling and symptomatic COPD.

Even when a smoker has developed symptomatic disease, stopping smoking will still result in worthwhile salvage of lung function and improved life expectancy. The main message for patients is:

It is never too late to stop!

Increasing age

COPD is a slowly progressive disorder, so increasing age is another risk factor. Symptoms appearing in someone under the age of 40 years should be regarded with suspicion and investigated fully because COPD is unlikely to be the cause, unless the sufferer is deficient in alpha-1 antitrypsin (α_1-AT). This is discussed in more detail later.

Gender

COPD is currently more common in men than women in the UK. A 1997 study of physician-diagnosed COPD showed a prevalence rate of:

- 1.7% of men,

- 1.4% of women.

However, the bad news is that, although the prevalence increased in men by 25% between 1990 and 1997, the increase in women during the same period was 69%. In men the prevalence of COPD levelled out in the mid-1990s but is continuing to rise in women.

It is also well recognised that physician-diagnosed COPD rates are an under-estimate of the true prevalence. A national study of ventilatory function in British adults in the mid-1980s – probably a truer picture of the prevalence of COPD – found reductions in lung function in the following proportions of people aged 40–65 years:

- 18% of male smokers,

- 7% of male non-smokers,

- 14% of female smokers,

- 6% of female non-smokers.

A population study from the USA, conducted in the mid-1990s, supports this earlier British study. It found prevalence rates of airflow limitation in white males of:

- 14.2% of current smokers,

- 6.9% of ex-smokers,

- 3.3% of non-smokers.

In white females the rates were:

- 13.6% of current smokers,

- 6.8% of ex-smokers,

- 3.1% of non-smokers.

These differences between male and female smokers might be related to the fact that in this age cohort smoking was more common in men than in women. With the increase in the number of women smokers, the preponderance of males is changing. Some recent work has suggested that female smokers are at even greater risk of developing COPD than their male counterparts.

Airway hyper-responsiveness

Airway hyper-responsiveness (AHR) has been proposed as a risk factor for the development of COPD. Certainly AHR is not the sole preserve of the person with asthma. It has been demonstrated extensively in smokers. Smokers also have raised levels of IgE, the antibody associated with atopy and asthma.

This observation forms the basis of the so-called Dutch hypothesis. Some doctors in the Netherlands have long regarded COPD and asthma as two aspects of the same process, and believe that at-risk smokers share an 'allergic' constitution that, when combined with smoking, is expressed as COPD. However, this hypothesis is controversial and it has been argued that raised levels of IgE and increased AHR in COPD patients could be the *result* of smoking rather than a pre-existing factor.

Lower socio-economic status

The prevalence of COPD is highest among people in lower socio-economic groups. Smoking rates are higher in these groups, but this may not be the sole causative factor.

Low birth weight is associated with a reduced FEV_1 in adult life. Airways develop in the first 16 weeks of gestation, and alveoli mature and increase in number in the last six weeks of gestation and first three years of life. The number of alveoli reaches adult levels of about 300 million by the age of 8 years. Thus, malnutrition of the fetus and serious lower respiratory tract infection (LRTI) in infancy during these periods of lung development may result in lung function failing to reach full potential. This may be an independent risk factor for reduced lung function in adult life and increased risk of COPD.

Maternal smoking has been extensively linked with low birth weight and recurrent LRTI in infancy, as have poor housing and social deprivation.

Poor diet

It has been suggested that antioxidants in the diet protect against the harmful effects of smoking and that a low dietary intake of antioxidant vitamins, such as vitamin C, is associated with decreased lung function and increased risk of COPD. Poor diet is also associated with socio-economic deprivation.

Occupation

Certain jobs have been linked with COPD. Coal mining is probably the most well-recognised occupational risk factor, but cotton processing, farming and other dusty occupations may also be relevant, particularly when added to the effects of smoking. Welding fumes are highly toxic, and welding, particularly in confined spaces, is suspected of being a risk factor. However, in the UK at present the only occupational cause of COPD for which compensation may be paid is coal mining.

Air pollution

Air pollution is often blamed by COPD sufferers for their disease. Before the Clean Air Acts of the 1950s, urban dwelling was associated with an increased risk: the air was polluted with heavy particles, soot and sulphur oxides. The pollution now experienced is mainly from vehicle exhaust emissions and photochemical pollutants such as ozone, produced by the action of sunlight on exhaust fumes. It is seldom disputed that these are respiratory irritants and that episodes of high pollution are associated with increased hospital admissions for respiratory problems. The role of these irritants *as a cause* of COPD, however, is more controversial. Nowadays, urban dwelling in the UK does not seem to pose a greater risk of COPD than rural dwelling.

Outdoor and indoor air pollution may, however, be significant in Third World countries. Indoor air pollution from biomass fuels, such as charcoal burned for cooking and heating, may carry a risk for the development of COPD.

Deficiency of alpha-1 antitrypsin

A rare, but well-recognised, risk factor for COPD is the inherited deficiency of alpha-1 antitrypsin. This is a protective enzyme that counteracts the destructive action of proteolytic enzymes in the lung. Deficiency of it is associated with the early development – between the ages of 20 and 40 years – of severe emphysema (see also the section 'Emphysema', below). The deficiency is inherited in a homozygous fashion with a frequency of 1:4000 of the population. Both parents will be carriers but the possession of a single abnormal chromosome does not seem to cause severe disease. There is usually a strong family history of COPD. Family members should be tested for alpha-1 antitrypsin deficiency and, if affected, must be very strongly advised never to smoke.

Genetics

Alpha-1 antitrypsin deficiency is an extensively studied genetic risk factor for COPD. It is now believed that many other genetic factors increase (and decrease) an individual's risk of developing COPD. Why there seem to be familial clusters of COPD cases and why some smokers develop COPD and others do not has intrigued many researchers. The genetics of COPD is being investigated intensively.

Chronic asthma

Asthma is defined as:

> 'a chronic inflammatory condition of the airways . . . in susceptible individuals inflammatory symptoms are usually associated with widespread, but variable, airflow obstruction and an increase in airway response to a variety of stimuli. Obstruction is often reversible, either spontaneously or with treatment.'

Long-standing asthma may result in permanent damage to the airways and subsequent loss of that reversibility. Long-standing bronchial hyper-reactivity can cause hypertrophy of the bronchial smooth muscle, just as skeletal muscles will hypertrophy if exercised regularly. Chronic epithelial disruption may result in the deposition of collagen in the basement membrane and fibrosis of the submucosal layer. The end result is a narrowed and distorted airway that can no longer bronchodilate fully.

The duration and severity of the asthma are risk factors for the development of fixed airflow obstruction. Approximately 1 in 10 people with early-onset asthma will develop a degree of fixed airflow obstruction; for those with late-onset asthma the proportion is higher – around 1 in 4. Smoking considerably increases this risk.

Recent studies have suggested that early intervention with inhaled steroids reduces the risk. Work in children with persistent asthma has shown that a two-year delay in introducing inhaled steroids results in a reduced potential for the lung function to improve, compared with the improvement found in children who commenced inhaled steroids immediately. Further work with adults has shown similar results, suggesting that early diagnosis and early, aggressive treatment with inhaled steroids may reduce the risk of long-term chronic airflow obstruction. There are also implications for ensuring that patients adhere to the therapy they are prescribed and don't smoke.

Occupational asthma – particularly if the diagnosis is delayed and exposure prolonged – can lead to chronic persistent symptoms and fixed airflow obstruction, even after the patient is removed from the offending occupational sensitiser.

Chronic bronchitis

Chronic bronchitis is defined by the Medical Research Council as:

> 'The production of sputum on most days for at least three months in at least two consecutive years.'

This definition describes a set of symptoms that are extremely common, if not universal, among long-term smokers and widely recognised as the 'smoker's cough'. Not all smokers whose illness fits the definition of chronic bronchitis will have an accelerated decline in lung function; 80% of smokers do not, after all, develop COPD. However, the GOLD guidelines suggest that those with a persistent cough and sputum production and a history of exposure to risk factors should be considered 'at risk' and should be tested for airflow obstruction even if they do not complain of breathlessness.

Recent research from the Netherlands has supported this suggestion. Random testing of smokers aged between 35 and 70 years revealed a reduced FEV_1 in 18% of all smokers. The percentage with a reduced FEV_1 rose to 27% in smokers with cough and to 48% of smokers over 60 years who also had a cough.

Mucus in the airways is produced by mucus glands, situated

mainly in the larger airways, and by goblet cells, found mainly in the lining of the smaller airways. Mucus glands produce about 40 times more mucus than the goblet cells, and it may be that the excess mucus production in smokers not affected by progressive airflow obstruction reflects changes in the large airways. This chronic hyper-secretion of mucus with little airflow obstruction, in the absence of other reasons for chronic mucus production such as bronchiectasis, is known as 'simple bronchitis'. However, in at-risk smokers who are developing chronic airflow obstruction, excess mucus production seems to accelerate the rate of decline of their lung function.

Chronic production of mucus is unpleasant and may predispose the sufferer to lower respiratory tract infection, but on its own is not thought to be universally associated with the development of airflow obstruction. Excess production of mucus ceases in the majority of smokers when they stop smoking, although an initial short-term increase is a common experience in smokers when they quit.

Emphysema

Emphysema is defined in structural and pathological terms as:

> 'A condition of the lung characterised by abnormal, permanent enlargement of the air spaces distal to the terminal bronchiole, accompanied by destruction of their walls.'

This definition describes a destructive process that is largely associated with cigarette smoking. Cigarette smoke is an irritant and results in low-grade inflammation of the airways and alveoli. Broncho-alveolar lavage of smokers' lungs reveals increased numbers of inflammatory cells, notably macrophages and neutrophils. These inflammatory cells produce elastases – proteolytic enzymes that destroy elastin, the protein that makes up lung tissue. In health, these enzymes are neutralised by anti-elastases, anti-proteolytic enzymes, the most widely studied of which is alpha-1 antitrypsin. Figures 2.3 and 2.4 show the histology of normal lung tissue and of emphysema.

Alpha-1 antitrypsin deficiency accounts for 1–2% of all cases of diagnosed COPD. It provides a good model for our current under-standing of the role of elastases and anti-elastases in the development of emphysema.

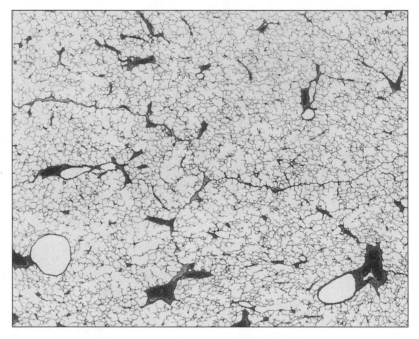

Figure 2.3 The histology of normal lung tissue

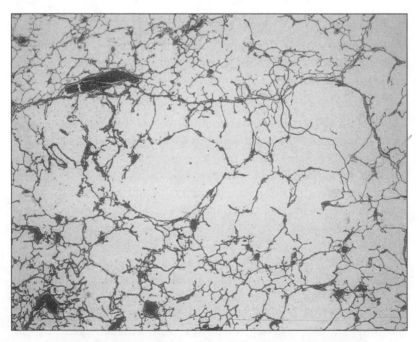

Figure 2.4 The histology of lung affected by emphysema

In early experiments, elastases introduced into lung tissue deficient in alpha-1 antitrypsin digested that lung tissue, thus producing emphysema. When alpha-1 antitrypsin was introduced into the deficient lung tissue – thereby effectively making it 'normal' – it protected against the action of the elastases and thus prevented emphysema.

That elastases are responsible for the destruction of lung tissue was confirmed by further experiments. A purified elastase was derived from neutrophils, a white blood cell attracted into the lungs of smokers. This neutrophil elastase (NE) was instilled into the lungs of experimental animals, causing a transient decrease in lung elastin, which then gradually returned to normal. However, although the loss of elastin was temporary, the structure of the animals' lungs was permanently damaged.

The elastase/anti-elastase hypothesis for the development of emphysema in humans is that the irritant effect of cigarette smoke increases the level of elastases in the lungs beyond the body's ability to neutralise them. Over many years lung elastin is lost, lung tissue is destroyed and emphysema results.

Although these and other experiments helped to explain the mechanisms behind the development of emphysema in people who are deficient in alpha-1 antitrypsin, it remains less clear what happens in people who are not deficient in this anti-proteolytic enzyme. There are several theories but further investigation is needed.

One theory is that, in some smokers, excessive numbers of inflammatory cells are attracted into the lungs in response to the irritant effects of cigarette smoke. These inflammatory cells, particularly neutrophils, are responsible for the release of elastases into the lung tissue; if too many are attracted into the lung, the amount of elastase they produce may outstrip the protective capacity of the anti-elastases. It is thought that in some individuals the inflammatory cells themselves produce excessive amounts of elastases.

Yet another hypothesis is that there is excessive inactivation of the protective anti-elastases such that the individual is somewhat deficient in these protective enzymes. It is thought that this inactivation may be caused by oxidants that are both present in cigarette smoke and released from the activated inflammatory cells present in the airways of smokers.

These hypotheses can be summarised as:

■ Abnormally high numbers of inflammatory cells are attracted into the airways, resulting in excessive production of elastases.

■ The inflammatory cells in the airways produce abnormally large amounts of elastases.

■ Oxidants found in cigarette smoke and released from inflammatory cells inactivate the protective anti-elastases in the lung.

In practice, all these mechanisms may be interacting in a single individual.

Elastases, NE in particular, have been implicated in the development of chronic bronchitis as well as emphysema. They have been found to produce an increase in the number of goblet cells, a feature of chronic bronchitis. NE is also a potent inducer of mucus secretion, and causes a reduction of ciliary beat frequency.

Thus elastase/anti-elastase imbalance may be implicated not only in the development of emphysema but also in the pathogenesis of chronic bronchitis.

Small airways disease

Cigarette smoking may result in pathological changes in the small airways as well as the alveoli. Structural changes in the small airways 2–5mm in diameter have been found in young smokers who have died suddenly from causes other than respiratory disease. Cigarette smoke causes chronic inflammation in the airways and repeated cycles of inflammation and repair. This leads to remodelling of the tissues of the airways. The changes include:

■ inflammation and oedema,

■ fibrosis,

■ collagen deposition,

■ smooth muscle hypertrophy,

■ occlusion of airway with mucus.

As a result, the airway becomes narrowed and distorted, causing resistance to airflow. Unfortunately, there can be considerable change in these airways without giving rise to symptoms. Indeed, this level of the bronchial tree is often referred to as the 'silent area' of the lungs.

COPD – a mixed spectrum of diseases

Although we can recognise the pathological entities of chronic bronchitis, small airways disease and emphysema, it is usual, clinically, for COPD patients to have features of more than one.

Consequences

Narrowing of the bronchioles results in increased resistance to airflow. Loss of elastin in the alveolar walls in emphysema contributes to the collapse of the small airways. The lung parenchyma is made up of the walls of alveoli, which support the small airways in the same way that taut guy ropes hold open the walls of a tent. Destruction of the alveolar walls in emphysema means that this support is lost and the airways will tend to collapse (Figure 2.5). Airway collapse is exacerbated by forced exhalation, such as occurs on exercise, and air is trapped in the lungs. Patients with emphysema may naturally adopt a strategy that helps to 'splint' the airways open. 'Pursed-lip' breathing helps maintain air pressure in the small airways, preventing them from collapsing. Patients seem to be 'grabbing' air and 'paying it out' gently. It is a useful, though not universal, clinical sign.

The elastic walls of the alveoli provide some of the driving force behind exhalation. Loss of this elasticity causes the lungs to become 'floppy' and hyperinflated. Emphysematous lungs may be 2–3 litres bigger than normal, but most of this extra capacity is inaccessible. Hyperinflation causes the diaphragms to flatten and the accessory muscles of respiration are then used to aid respiration. The inefficient respiratory movements caused by hyperinflation lead to increased breathlessness on exertion, when the work of breathing is heightened and the respiratory rate is raised.

Loss of the alveolar/capillary interface causes disruption of gas exchange. The surface area for gas exchange in normal lungs is about the size of a tennis court. Emphysema reduces this area and thus

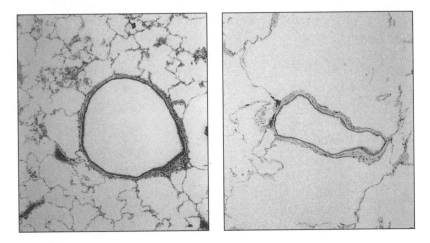

Figure 2.5 Histology showing the loss of the 'guy ropes', resulting in airway collapse

reduces the capacity to exchange oxygen and carbon dioxide in the lungs. In the early stages of the disease the body is able to compensate for this loss by increasing the respiratory drive. As the disease progresses, however, the ability to compensate successfully diminishes and the blood gases become persistently abnormal, with serious consequences.

When the respiratory drive is responsive, abnormalities of blood gases will result in an increase in both respiratory drive and respiratory rate. The blood gases will be normalised but the patient will be breathless. Eventually the progression of the disease overcomes the ability of even the most responsive respiratory drive to compensate, and respiratory failure ensues.

Breathlessness makes everyday activities such as shopping, cooking and eating difficult. Weight loss is common and is associated with a poor prognosis. Although it was originally thought that weight loss in COPD was due to a combination of increased expenditure of energy at rest because of the increased effort of breathing and of difficulty in maintaining an adequate energy intake, it is now recognised that this is unlikely to be the sole cause. Loss of lean body mass affects the ability to fight infection. Infective exacerbations may become more common and recovery will be slower. (Weight loss and nutrition are discussed in more detail in Chapter 9.)

Some patients seem to have a less responsive respiratory drive and, as the disease progresses, they will become unable to normalise their blood gases. They will be less breathless but will suffer from the long-term consequences of low levels of oxygen in the blood (hypoxia), cor pulmonale, pulmonary hypertension and polycythaemia.

Cor pulmonale is a complex and incompletely understood syndrome of fluid retention and pulmonary hypertension caused by chronic **hypoxia**. The kidneys are affected by hypoxia, causing renin–angiotensin upset. This results in fluid retention and peripheral oedema.

Polycythaemia A way for the body to adapt to chronic hypoxia is to produce more haemoglobin to carry what little oxygen is available, increasing the number of erythrocytes and raising the packed cell volume (haematocrit). However, this predisposes an already less mobile patient to deep vein thrombosis and pulmonary embolism.

Pulmonary hypertension When areas of the lung are poorly ventilated – ventilation/perfusion mismatch – the alveolar capillary bed becomes constricted, causing increased pressure in the pulmonary vasculature – pulmonary hypertension. For a simplistic but helpful analogy for hypoxic pulmonary capillary constriction, imagine the lungs as a railway station. To work efficiently, passengers (*oxygen*) must reach the platforms (*alveoli*) where the trains (*blood supply*) can pick them up. If the passengers cannot reach the platforms (*poor ventilation*), the trains will go away empty and the railway system will be inefficient (*ventilation/perfusion mismatch*). If this situation persists, the railway line will be shut down (*pulmonary capillary constriction*). Eventually the track will be lifted so that, even if the passengers do reach the platform, the trains will no longer be there to pick them up. (*Structural changes in the blood vessel walls eventually result in irreversible capillary constriction.*)

The right ventricle has to work harder to pump an increased circulating volume of blood through a disrupted and constricted capillary bed. Initially it will enlarge to compensate for the extra workload, but will eventually fail, increasing the peripheral oedema. Clinically, cor pulmonale resembles right ventricular failure but, at least to begin with, the right ventricle may be functioning reasonably well.

The clinical pictures described above are recognisable as the 'pink puffer' and the 'blue bloater', but such terminology is currently out of favour and may not be particularly helpful. In practice the picture is less clear and patients often cannot be placed neatly into one or other category. Suffice it to say that some patients with appalling lung function and intolerable breathlessness will struggle on with reasonable blood gases whilst others, with less severely impaired lung function, will develop oedema and cor pulmonale relatively early. Intermittent ankle oedema and central cyanosis are a poor prognostic sign. Untreated, the three-year survival of such patients is only 30%. Long-term oxygen therapy (LTOT) can increase survival considerably; it is covered in detail in Chapter 9.

Further reading

Risk factors

AGERTOFT L, PEDERSEN S (1994) Effects of long-term treatment with an inhaled corticosteroid on growth and pulmonary function in asthmatic children. *Respiratory Medicine* **88**: 373–81

BARKER DJP, GODFREY KM, FALL C et al. (1991) Relation of birth weight and childhood respiratory infection to adult lung function and death from chronic obstructive lung disease. *British Medical Journal* **303**: 671–5

BUIST AS, VOLLMER WM (1994) Smoking and other risk factors. In: Murray JF, Nadel JA (eds) *Textbook of Respiratory Medicine*. WB Saunders, Philadelphia PA; 1259–87

COX BD (1987) Blood pressure and respiratory function. In: *The Health and Lifestyle Survey. Preliminary report of a nationwide survey of the physical and mental health, attitudes and lifestyle of a random sample of 9003 British adults*. Health Promotion Research Trust, London; 17–33

FLETCHER C, PETO R (1977) The natural history of chronic airflow obstruction. *British Medical Journal* **1**: 1645–8

HAAHTELA T, JARVINEN M, KAVA T et al. (1994) Effects of reducing or discontinuing inhaled budesonide in patients with mild asthma. *New England Journal of Medicine* **331**: 700–5

LEBOWITZ M (1977) Occupational exposures in relation to symptomatology and lung function in a community population. *Environmental Research* **44**: 59–67

LEBOWITZ MD (1996) Epidemiological studies of the respiratory effects of air pollution. *American Journal of Respiratory and Critical Care Medicine* **9**: 1029–54

MANN SL, WADSWORTH MEJ, COLLEY JRT (1992) Accumulation of factors influencing respiratory illness in members of a national birth cohort and their offspring. *Journal of Epidemiology and Community Health* **46**: 286–92

O'CONNOR GT, SPARROW D, WEISS ST (1989) The role of allergy and non-specific airway hyperresponsiveness in the pathogenesis of chronic obstructive pulmonary disease. *American Review of Respiratory Disease* **140**: 225–52

SCHWARTZ J, WEISS ST (1990) Dietary factors and their relation to respiratory symptoms. *American Journal of Epidemiology* **132**: 67–76

SILVERMAN EK, SPEIZER FE (1996) Risk factors for the development of chronic obstructive pulmonary disease. *Medical Clinics of North America* **80**: 501–22

SORIANO JR, MAIER WC, EGGER P et al. (2000) Recent trends in physician diagnosed COPD in men and women in the UK. *Thorax* **55**: 789–94

VAN SCHAYCK CP, LOOZEN JMC, WAGENA E (2002) Detecting patients at high risk of developing chronic obstructive pulmonary disease in general practice: a cross-sectional case-finding study. *British Medical Journal* **324**: 1370–4

Pathology

MACNEE W (1995) Pulmonary circulation, cardiac function and fluid balance. In: Calverley P, Pride N (eds) *Chronic Obstructive Pulmonary Disease*. Chapman and Hall Medical, London; 243–91

PETO R, SPEIZER FE, MOORE CF et al. (1983) The relevance in adults of airflow obstruction, but not of mucous hypersecretion in mortality from chronic lung disease. *American Review of Respiratory Disease* **128**: 491–500

STOCKLEY RA (1995) Biochemical and cellular mechanisms. In: Calverley P, Pride N (eds) *Chronic Obstructive Pulmonary Disease*. Chapman and Hall Medical, London; 93–133

3 Presentation and history

Main points

1 COPD is rare in someone who has never smoked or is a genuinely light smoker.

2 A significant smoking history for COPD is more than 15–20 pack-years.

3 The commonest and most distressing symptom of COPD is breathlessness on exertion.

4 Symptoms are slowly progressive and non-variable.

5 COPD patients are generally not woken at night by their symptoms.

6 A previous history of asthma, atopic illness or childhood chestiness may point to a diagnosis of asthma rather than COPD.

7 Clinical signs of COPD are generally not apparent until the disease is severe.

8 Clinical signs in severe disease include:
   – Barrel chest
   – Prominent accessory muscles of respiration
   – Recession of lower costal margins
   – Abdominal breathing
   – Weight loss
   – Central cyanosis
   – Peripheral oedema
   – Raised jugular venous pressure

9 Alternative diagnoses must be carefully considered and excluded.

Symptoms

The most common presenting symptoms of COPD are breathlessness on exertion and cough, with or without sputum production. However, considerable loss of lung function can occur before symptoms become apparent, with the result that patients frequently consult their GP only when the disease is at an advanced stage. COPD is a slowly progressive disorder and patients gradually adapt their lives to their disability, not noticing breathlessness until it is severe enough to have a significant impact on their ability to perform everyday tasks. Most smokers expect to cough and be short of breath, and they often dismiss the symptoms of progressive airflow obstruction as a normal consequence of their smoking habit. A smokers' cough, far from being a harmless, insignificant consequence of smoking, is often an early warning sign of COPD.

Breathlessness

The most important and common symptom in COPD, 'breathlessness' is a subjective term. It can be defined as an awareness of increased or inappropriate respiratory effort. Patients describe breathlessness in different ways, but the person with COPD will frequently describe it as difficulty inhaling:

'I just can't get enough air in!'

In health the increased oxygen demand that occurs with exercise is met by using some of the inspiratory reserve volume of the lungs to increase the tidal volume (see Figure 4.11). In COPD, because the calibre of the airways is relatively fixed, the inspiratory reserve volume cannot be fully used. Hyperinflation of the lungs with air-trapping in the alveoli leads to increased residual volume at the expense of inspiratory reserve volume, thus worsening breathlessness. Dynamic airway collapse due to loss of the 'guy ropes' (see Chapter 2) in emphysema causes further air-trapping, adding to the residual volume and increasing breathlessness on exertion. Flattening of the diaphragms when the lungs are hyperinflated means that the accessory muscles of respiration become increasingly important. Any activity, such as carrying shopping or stretching up, that uses these muscles for activities other than breathing will worsen breathlessness. COPD patients often also find it difficult to bend forward, for example to tie shoelaces.

Loss of the alveolar/capillary interface in COPD also means that the increased demand for oxygen that activity imposes cannot be met, and this also increases the sensation of breathlessness.

In asthma, breathlessness is variable; in COPD, it varies little from day to day. The answer to the question 'Do you have good days and bad days?' can thus be illuminating. The other major differences between the breathlessness of COPD and the breathlessness of asthma are that the patient with COPD is rarely woken at night by the symptoms and, until the disease is very severe, is not breathless at rest.

Although breathlessness is slowly progressive, patients will often relate the onset of symptoms to a recent event, notably a chest infection, and will claim to have 'Never been the same since then'. Close questioning will often reveal that the problem is indeed long-standing but that patients have unconsciously adapted their lifestyle to fit the disability. They will perhaps have avoided talking while walking, walked slower than their peers or have started to take the car when they would previously have walked. The chest infection was simply the 'straw that broke the camel's back'.

Cough

A productive cough either precedes or appears simultaneously with the onset of breathlessness in 75% of COPD patients. The cough is usually worse in the mornings but, unlike the asthma patient, the patient with COPD is seldom woken at night. Morning cough and chest tightness are usually quickly relieved by expectoration. Indeed, many patients justify the first cigarette of the day because it helps them to 'clear the tubes'. Morning symptoms in asthma frequently last for several hours.

Sputum

The production of sputum is a common, though not universal, feature of COPD. It is usually white or grey, but may become mucopurulent, green or yellow with exacerbations. It is generally less tenacious and 'tacky' than the sputum in asthma. Excessive production (half a cup full or more) of sputum and frequent infective episodes should raise the possibility of bronchiectasis, and any report of haemoptysis must be taken seriously. You should refer the patient immediately for chest x-ray and a consultant's opinion, because COPD patients have a high incidence of bronchial carcinoma.

The production of copious amounts of frothy sputum, particularly if it is associated with orthopnoea or a previous history of hypertension or ischaemic heart disease, may raise suspicions of left ventricular failure and pulmonary oedema.

Wheezing

Wheeze is a common presenting symptom in both COPD and asthma. COPD patients commonly experience wheeze when walking 'into the wind' or going out into cold air. Unlike people with asthma, they are rarely wheezy at rest and are not woken at night by wheeze. The atopic asthmatic will often relate wheezing episodes to exposure to a specific allergen.

History taking

COPD is unusual in a non-smoker, so it is important to quantify an individual's exposure to cigarettes as accurately as possible in terms of 'pack-years'. Smoking 20 cigarettes a day (a pack) for a year equates to one pack-year, 10 a day for a year is one-half pack-year, 40 a day for a year is two pack-years . . . and so on. The formula is:

$$\frac{\text{Number smoked per day}}{20} \times \text{Number of years smoked}$$

For example, if a patient smoked 10 cigarettes a day from the age of 14 years to 20 years, that is

$$\frac{10}{20} \times 6 = 3 \text{ pack-years}$$

When doing national service he started smoking seriously! – 20 a day until 45 years of age. That is:

$$\frac{20}{20} \times 25 = 25 \text{ pack-years}$$

Then he made a real effort to cut down and managed to get down to 5 a day until he finally stopped smoking aged 57 years:

$$\frac{5}{20} \times 12 = 3 \text{ pack-years}$$

It is therefore possible to calculate this patient's total cigarette exposure as

$$3 + 25 + 3 = 31 \text{ pack-years}.$$

A significant smoking history for COPD is more than 15–20 pack-years. If the smoking history is genuinely light, you should look carefully and exhaustively for other causes for the symptoms.

Any exposure to organic dusts, coal dust or welding fumes may be significant, so it is important to find out about a patient's occupational history. Bear in mind, too, that previous jobs might have exposed the patient to agents that could cause persistent, severe, occupational asthma.

It is important to establish when the symptoms started. 'Chestiness' in childhood might have been undiagnosed asthma that has recurred in adult life. Any family history of asthma or a previous history of atopic illness may point to a likelihood of asthma rather than COPD.

Smoking predisposes the patient to ischaemic heart disease as well as to COPD, and many older patients will be receiving treatment for hypertension. A full medical history and current drug therapy may highlight the possibility of a cardiac cause for the patient's symptoms.

Excluding other possible causes of breathlessness is very important. (Assessment and differential diagnosis are covered in detail in Chapters 4 and 5.)

Clinical signs

In mild and moderate disease, clinical signs are mostly absent. It is not until the disease is severe that clinical signs become apparent. *Early COPD is detectable only by measuring lung function with a spirometer.* (Spirometry is discussed in Chapter 4.) More can be gained by inspecting the chest than by examining it with a stethoscope. Removing the patient's shirt and taking a good look can be most informative. Although a definitive diagnosis does not depend on the examination alone, it is still an essential part of the assessment and can be used to support the history and the diagnostic tests. In severe disease the chest may be hyperinflated, with an increased anteroposterior diameter and a typical 'barrel' shape. The ribs become more horizontal and, because the position of the trachea is fixed by the mediastinum, the trachea may look shortened – the distance between the cricoid cartilage and the xiphisternal notch will be less than three finger-breadths. The trachea may also seem to be being pulled downwards with each breath.

Chest percussion may reveal that the liver is displaced downwards by the flattened diaphragms. Relatively quiet vesicular breath sounds may be heard on auscultation. Wheeze may also be audible, as may râles, particularly at the lung bases.

The strap muscles of the neck may be prominent and the lower intercostal margins drawn in on inhalation (Hoover's sign). Use of the abdominal muscles to aid exhalation may also be apparent, although movements of the rib cage during respiration may be relatively small. The angle between the lower ribs and the sternum – the xiphisternal angle – may widen because the rib cage is raised due to hyperinflation of the lungs. Flattening of the diaphragm may also displace the contents of the abdomen forward, giving the patient a pot-bellied appearance.

In severe disease the effort of walking into the consulting room and undressing will be sufficient to make most patients breathless, and the fact that breathing is hard work will be immediately obvious. They may lean forward, shoulders raised, resting their arms on the table to ease their breathing. Their respiratory rate will be raised and they may use 'pursed-lip' breathing. Their speech may be somewhat 'staccato' because they will not be able to complete a sentence without stopping for breath, and exhalation may be prolonged.

In patients with cor pulmonale the jugular venous pressure (JVP) will be raised, and there will be ankle oedema and central cyanosis. All of these are poor prognostic signs and must be taken seriously. Abnormal blood gases may be associated with loss of mental agility and the ability to concentrate. Elevated carbon dioxide may cause drowsiness and mental confusion, and a typical 'flapping' tremor of the hands when the arms are outstretched.

Finger clubbing is not a feature of COPD but may suggest bronchiectasis or a pulmonary tumour. Weight loss is common in advanced COPD, and another poor prognostic sign. Because malignancy is also a cause of weight loss in this group of middle-aged to elderly smokers, this must be excluded.

Summary

COPD presents as a slowly progressive, non-variable disease that causes breathlessness on exertion and cough with or without the production of sputum. The disease eventually affects every aspect of a patient's life and causes significant disability and handicap. Generally, clinical signs are apparent only when the disease is advanced, and the detection of early disease relies on a high level of suspicion about respiratory symptoms in patients who smoke and the referral of such patients for spirometry.

Further reading

CALVERLEY PMA, GEORGOPOULOS D (1998) Chronic obstructive pulmonary disease: symptoms and signs. In: Postma DS, Siafakis NM (eds) *Management of Chronic Obstructive Pulmonary Disease. European Respiratory Monograph:* **3** (May): 6–24

PEARSON MG, CALVERLEY PMA (1995) Clinical and laboratory assessment. In: Calverley P, Pride N (eds) *Chronic Obstructive Pulmonary Disease.* Chapman and Hall Medical, London; 309–49

4 Spirometry and lung function tests

Main points

1 Spirometry measures airflow and lung volumes, and is the preferred lung function test in COPD.

2 The forced vital capacity (FVC) is the total volume of air that can be exhaled with maximum force, starting from maximum inhalation and continuing to maximum exhalation.

3 The forced expiratory volume in one second (FEV_1) is the amount of air that can be exhaled in the first second of a forced blow from maximum inhalation.

4 Both the FVC and the FEV_1 are expressed as volumes (in litres) and as a percentage of the predicted values. Predicted values have been determined from large population studies, and are dependent on age, height, gender and ethnicity.

5 The ratio of FEV_1 to FVC (FEV_1/FVC) is expressed as a percentage. Values of less than 70% indicate airflow obstruction.

6 In diseases that cause airflow obstruction the FEV_1 will be below 80% of the predicted value and the FEV_1/FVC ratio will be less than 70%. (In severe COPD the FVC may also be less than 80% of predicted.)

7 In restrictive lung diseases both the FEV_1 and the FVC will be below 80% of the predicted value but the FEV_1/FVC ratio will be normal or high.

8 The volume/time trace must be smooth, upward and free of irregularities. The graph must reach a plateau, demonstrating that the patient has blown to FVC.

9 The forced expiratory manoeuvre can also be presented as graphs of flow rate against volume – the flow/volume trace. They show airflow through small airways and can be particularly useful in detecting early airflow obstruction.

10 Further tests, such as a gas transfer test (TLco) and static lung volumes, are available in lung function laboratories, and may be helpful.

11 Training in the proper use and interpretation of spirometry is essential.

Measuring lung function to determine the presence and severity of airflow obstruction in COPD is as fundamental as measuring blood pressure to detect and monitor hypertension.

The preferred and recommended lung function test is spirometry, which provides indices not only of airflow but also of lung volume. Since the publication of the BTS *COPD Guidelines*, general practices have been encouraged to obtain a spirometer. To benefit fully from its use, both doctors and practice nurses need training to understand the blowing technique and the interpretation of results. An alternative to having a spirometer in the practice may be open access spirometry at the local respiratory unit.

Spirometry

What does it mean?

In simple terms, spirometry measures two parameters – **airflow** from fully inflated lungs and the **total volume** of air that can be exhaled from maximum inhalation to maximum exhalation, using maximum force to blow all the air out as hard and as fast as possible. In a healthy individual this forced expiratory manoeuvre can normally be completed in three to four seconds, but with increasing airflow obstruction it takes longer to push all the air out of the lungs. In severe COPD it may take up to 15 seconds.

The volume of air exhaled is plotted on a graph against the time taken to reach maximum exhalation. Volume is plotted on the x (vertical) axis, and time on the y (horizontal) axis. This is known as the volume/time trace. Three indices can be derived from this trace:

1 FEV_1 – the forced expired volume in the first second.

2 FVC – the total volume of air that can be exhaled from maximal inhalation to maximal exhalation (the forced vital capacity).

3 FEV_1/FVC% – the ratio of FEV_1 to FVC, expressed as a percentage.

The FEV_1 and FVC are expressed in absolute values in litres and also as a percentage of the predicted values for that individual, depending on their age, height, gender and ethnic origin. For example, the predicted (mean) level of FEV_1 for a 30-year-old white male 1.70 metres tall is 3.86 litres and for a 65-year-old woman 1.50 metres tall it is 1.7 litres, based on a European Respiratory Society population survey conducted in 1993. Readings 20% either side of the predicted value are considered to be within the normal range. Thus an FEV_1 or FVC over 80% of the predicted value is normal.

When the airways are normal, 70–85% of the total volume of air in the lungs (FVC) can be exhaled in the first second. In other words, the FEV_1 normally comprises 70–85% of the FVC; the ratio of the FEV_1 to the FVC (FEV_1/FVC) is 70–85%. This is calculated by dividing the patient's FEV_1 by their FVC and multiplying by 100. When airflow through the airways is obstructed, less air can be exhaled in the first second and the FEV_1/FVC ratio falls. Levels below 70% indicate airflow obstruction. Examples of calculating lung function are given in Table 4.1.

Table 4.1 Calculating lung function in normal and obstructed patterns

Normal	*Obstructed*
FEV_1 = 3.0 litres	FEV_1 = 1.8 litres
FVC = 4.0 litres	FVC = 3.8 litres
FEV_1/FVC% = $\dfrac{3.0}{4.0} \times 100$	FEV_1/FVC% = $\dfrac{1.8}{3.8} \times 100$
= 75%	= 47%

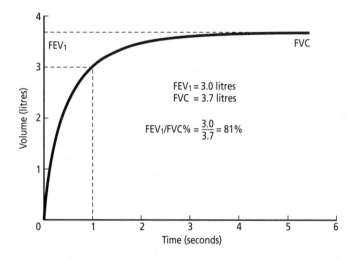

Figure 4.1 Normal spirometry (volume/time trace)

The shape of the volume/time trace should be smooth and convex upwards, and achieve a satisfactory plateau indicating that exhalation is complete (Figure 4.1). The FEV_1 is very reproducible and varies by less than 120ml between blows if the test is carried out correctly. The FVC can show more variation, as it will depend on how hard the subject tries to blow the last remaining air out of the lungs.

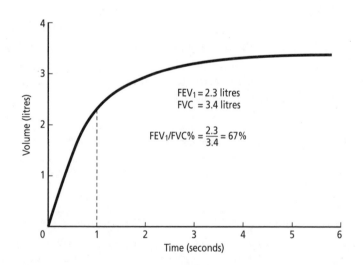

Figure 4.2 Mild obstruction

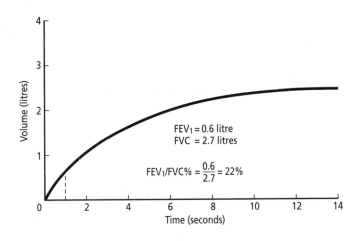

Figure 4.3 Severe obstruction

Another extra manoeuvre, in addition to the forced expiratory manoeuvre discussed above, is the relaxed or slow vital capacity (VC), in which the patient blows out at their own pace after maximal inhalation. This can be useful in COPD; if the airways are unsupported, they might collapse during a forced blow. In COPD, the VC is often 0.5 litre greater than the FVC.

Obstructive pattern

With increasing airflow obstruction it takes longer to exhale and the early slope of the volume/time trace becomes less steep. Figures 4.2 and 4.3 show examples of mild and more severe obstruction. The FEV_1 is reduced both as a volume and as a percentage of the predicted value. The FEV_1/FVC likewise falls. The FVC in COPD and asthma is usually better maintained at near-normal levels until airflow obstruction is severe.

Restrictive pattern

Spirometry is helpful in the assessment of other respiratory conditions. In patients with, for example, lung scarring, diffuse fibrosis, pleural effusions or rib cage deformity the lung volumes become reduced. Airway size remains normal, which means that air can be blown out at the normal rate. This produces a trace (Figure 4.4) with

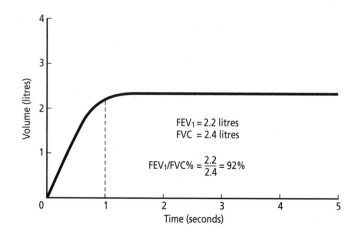

$$FEV_1 = 2.2 \text{ litres}$$
$$FVC = 2.4 \text{ litres}$$

$$FEV_1/FVC\% = \frac{2.2}{2.4} = 92\%$$

Figure 4.4 Restrictive defect

a normal-shaped volume/time curve and a normal FEV_1/FVC ratio. The values of FEV_1 and FVC are reduced. This is called a restrictive pattern. Peak expiratory flow (PEF, see below) in such patients is normal.

Table 4.2 summarises the values for FEV_1, FVC, FEV_1/FVC ratio and PEF in normal, obstructive and restrictive patterns. Table 4.3 categorises the conditions likely to be causing obstructive or restrictive disease.

Table 4.2 Summary of values for FEV_1, FVC, FEV_1/FVC ratio and PEF in normal, obstructive and restrictive patterns

	Normal	*Obstruction*	*Restriction*
FVC	above 80% predicted	above 80% predicted	below 80% predicted
FEV_1	above 80% predicted	below 80% predicted	below 80% predicted
FEV_1/FVC	above 70%	below 70%	above 70% (or high)
PEF	above 85% predicted	below 85% predicted	above 85% predicted

Table 4.3 Summary of likely conditions causing obstructive or restrictive disease

Obstructive disease	Restrictive disease
Generalised obstruction	Sarcoid
Asthma	Fibrosing alveolitis
COPD	Extrinsic allergic alveolitis
Bronchiectasis	Malignant infiltration
Cystic fibrosis	Asbestosis
Obliterative bronchiolitis	Pleural effusions
	Kyphoscoliosis
Localised obstruction	Ascites
Tumour	Obesity
Inhalation of foreign body	
Post-tracheotomy stenosis	

Blowing technique and reproducibility

Preparing the patient

- The patient should be clinically stable (i.e. at least four weeks should have elapsed since the last exacerbation).

- The patient should not have taken a short-acting bronchodilator (beta-2 agonist or anticholinergic) in the last four to six hours. Long-acting inhaled beta-2 agonists (including combination products) should be withheld for 12 hours, tiotropium for 24 hours and sustained-release oral bronchodilators (theophyllines and oral beta-2 agonists) for 24 hours.

- The patient should be advised not to eat a large meal within two hours of the test and should avoid vigorous exercise 30 minutes before testing. He or she should be encouraged to arrive in plenty of time, to rest and relax prior to testing.

- The patient should not be wearing a corset or other restrictive clothing, and should remove any loose-fitting dentures or chewing gum.

- Ensure that the patient is comfortable; invite them to empty their bladder before proceeding.

Some patients find it very hard to do without their short-acting bronchodilators. If they are unable to do without for four to six hours, two hours' abstinence is acceptable. Repeat tests should be done under the same conditions, at the same time of day and by the same operator to ensure that results are comparable.

Blowing technique

- The patient should be sitting in an upright position (not standing, because there is a potential risk of their feeling faint or dizzy, especially after repeated blows).

- Explain and demonstrate the technique to the patient.

- Ask the patient to take a maximal breath in and then place their lips around the mouthpiece to form an airtight seal.

- Ask the patient to exhale as hard, fast and completely as possible (with lots of encouragement from you). In a healthy person it may take only three to four seconds to complete the blow. With increasing airflow obstruction, it becomes harder to blow air out rapidly and exhalation can take as long as 15 seconds.

- Allow the patient adequate time – including time for recovery between blows, with a maximum of eight forced manoeuvres in one session.

Technical standards

- Three technically satisfactory manoeuvres should be made, giving similar results (good reproducibility) (see Figure 4.5).

- The best two readings of FEV_1 and FVC should be within 100ml or 5% of each other.

Common faults

The most common faults are:

- stopping blowing too early,
- coughing during the blow,
- submaximal effort.

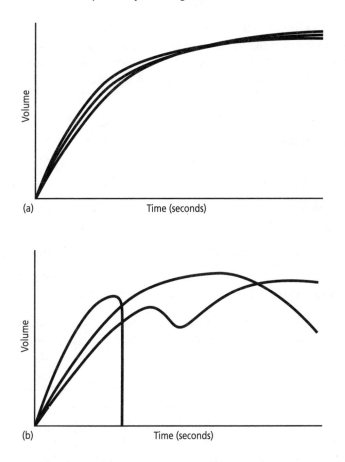

Figure 4.5 (a) Good reproducibility of blows; (b) poor reproducibility

Why is FEV₁ the preferred test?

The British, American, European and international COPD guide-lines all use FEV_1 as a percentage of predicted value as the basis for diagnosis and for estimating the severity of the disease. The new NICE Guidelines use the following scale:

- FEV_1 % predicted 50–80% – mild disease,
- FEV_1 % predicted 30–49% – moderate disease,
- FEV_1 % predicted below 30% – severe disease.

GOLD has also been changed, with FEV_1 and FEV_1/FVC ratio still determining the severity levels but these differ from NICE and the similar banding that is likely to be adopted by the American and European Respiratory Societies. For the latest GOLD severity banding, see Chapter 12.

The FEV_1 is the measurement of choice because:

- It is reproducible with well-defined normal ranges according to age, height, gender and ethnicity.

- It is quick and relatively easy to measure.

- Other diagnostic measurements such as FVC and FEV_1/FVC are recorded, which help in differential diagnosis.

- Variance of repeated measurements in any individual is low.

- FEV_1 predicts future mortality not only from COPD but also from other respiratory and cardiac disorders.

- FEV_1 is better related to prognosis and disability than FEV_1/FVC; this is mainly because the FVC, depending as it does on effort, is more variable.

The peak expiratory flow (PEF) measures the maximal flow rate that can be maintained over the first 10 milliseconds (ms) of a forced blow. It often under-estimates the degree of airflow obstruction in COPD, and the relationship between PEF and FEV_1 is poor. In milder COPD the PEF may be normal. (In asthma the correlation is better.)

Types of spirometer

Spirometers are essentially of two types:

- they measure volume directly (e.g. the dry bellows type of device),

- they measure flow through a pneumotachograph or turbine flowhead and electronically convert the values into volumes.

Electronic spirometers, which are mostly of the second type, usually have the facility to enter patient's age, height and gender, and will automatically calculate predicted values and the percentage of normal of the measured values. They have real-time traces of each blow, which can be superimposed on each other and the variance calculated to assist in assessing reproducibility. Many will also produce a flow/volume curve (see below) as well as the volume/time trace.

There are many effective spirometers, from the simple hand-held electronic device costing about £300 to more sophisticated equipment with many other facilities which can cost up to ten times that amount. Primary care needs are for simple, easy-to-use spirometers that preferably produce a hard copy printout of the trace and results. Some spirometers offer the facility for results and traces to be stored on a computer database. This type of equipment usually costs at least £1300. The low-cost hand-held devices do not allow a proper assessment of the quality or reproducibility of the procedure.

Nearly all spirometers require regular calibration checks with a 3-litre syringe but the manufacturers of some electronic devices claim that their instrument is accurate for at least three years without further calibration. The manufacturer's recommendations for servicing and calibration should be adhered to.

Training in the use of the spirometer and in the interpretation of results is essential. Courses for doctors and nurses are becoming increasingly available from official nurse training centres such as the National Respiratory Training Centre (NRTC) and from spirometer manufacturers. Training may also be available at local lung function centres, and the Association of Respiratory Technicians and Physiologists (an organisation affiliated to the British Thoracic Society) run independent training courses and assess and certify competence with the technique.

Lung age

Some electronic spirometers will calculate 'lung age' from the measured and predicted FEV_1. If the FEV_1 is reduced, this factor may be used to try to persuade patients to stop smoking – for example, knowing that their lung age is, say, 10–15 years greater than their actual age can be a powerful incentive.

Flow/volume measurement

Many modern spirometers measure a plot of expiratory flow rate throughout the entire expiratory blow, at the same time as the standard volume/time trace. A PEF, in contrast, measures only the

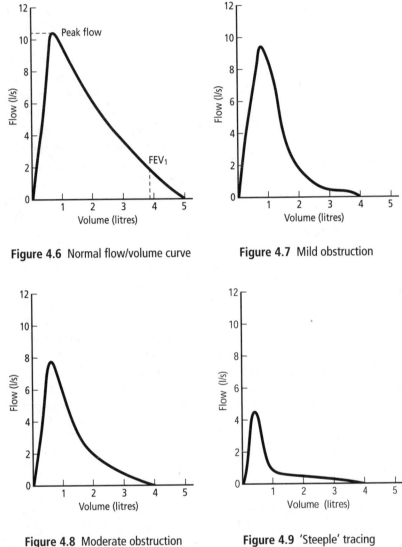

Figure 4.6 Normal flow/volume curve   **Figure 4.7** Mild obstruction

Figure 4.8 Moderate obstruction   **Figure 4.9** 'Steeple' tracing in severe emphysema

maximal flow rate that can be sustained for 10 milliseconds and represents flow only from the larger airways. The flow/volume trace, on the other hand, interprets flow from all generations of airways and is more helpful in detecting early narrowing in small airways, as in early COPD. It is also useful for differentiating between asthma and COPD, and can help to determine when there are mixed obstructive and restrictive defects.

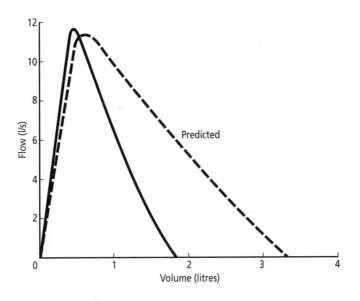

Figure 4.10 Restrictive pattern

For primary care purposes, interpretation need only extend to understanding the shape of the flow/volume curve. Figures 4.6, 4.7 and 4.8 give examples of normal, mild and moderate airflow obstruction. Figure 4.9 shows the classic 'steeple' pattern of airway collapse with emphysema, in which airways suddenly shut down on forced exhalation with low residual flow from the smaller airways. Figure 4.10 demonstrates the restrictive pattern with a normal shape curve and PEF but small FVC.

Other uses of spirometry

Measuring FEV_1 and FVC provides much more information than a simple PEF. Spirometers can therefore be useful in screening and following a whole range of respiratory disorders. The main areas of use are:

- obstructive lung disease,
- restrictive lung diseases,
- diagnosing and monitoring occupational lung disease,
- screening of smokers,

- medical examinations for scuba diving, aviation and insurance,

- health screening and possible screening of new patients (although the value of screening in asymptomatic non-smokers is controversial).

Early screening for COPD

In an ideal world, there might be advantages to screening populations at risk – smokers from about 35 years onwards – to detect early indications of airflow obstruction. This could be enhanced with a flow/volume trace, which is the most sensitive simple test for detecting early changes. In a recent study from the Netherlands, airflow obstruction was found in 27% of smokers with a cough.

Stopping patients smoking at this stage – admittedly not an easy task – would largely prevent COPD in most of them as well as reducing their risk of lung cancer and cardiovascular disease. There is some encouraging evidence from Poland that patients who are found to have airflow obstruction on general screening are more likely to stop smoking. In the long term there could be considerable cost saving for the nation. Unfortunately, there are not the money, time, resources and staff available to perform widespread screening at present.

Peak expiratory flow (PEF)

PEF is a simple, quick and inexpensive way of measuring airflow obstruction. It has been particularly useful in the diagnosis and monitoring of asthma.

The PEF meter measures the maximal flow rate that can be maintained over 10 milliseconds and usually detects a narrowing of large and medium-sized airways. It is most effective for monitoring changes in airflow in an individual over time. It has less value diagnostically because, as mentioned earlier, it may under-diagnose the severity of airflow obstruction in COPD.

The blowing technique requires the patient to inhale fully and then make a short maximal blow into the device (likened to blowing out candles on a birthday cake). The reading is expressed in litres per minute (l/min). It should be noted that, because the expiratory blowing technique is quite different from that required for spirometry, the readings for PEF will not be the same as those obtained from a peak flow meter. The reading from a PEF meter is usually greater by 50–100 litres per minute. The result from blowing into a PEF meter is less reproducible than with spirometry, and some patients use some very strange techniques for blowing – from a cough-like action to almost spitting into the device.

In the UK the scale on the peak flow instrument is linear. In most other countries around the world the mid range levels of the scale have been modified, making the readings non-linear and thus more accurate. This may not have any clinical bearing unless a patient is using different instruments with different scales. Home monitoring with one instrument is thus quite accurate and changes in PEF are clinically relevant, particularly in asthma care.

PEF can be helpful in COPD but should never be considered diagnostic or quantitative in terms of severity. It can be useful to perform twice-daily readings at home during a trial of an oral steroid or when it is uncertain whether the diagnosis is asthma or COPD.

Gas transfer test (TLco)

This very useful test is performed in hospital lung-function laboratories. The single-breath diffusion test measures the ability of the alveolar air/blood interface to transfer a trace amount of carbon monoxide into the pulmonary circulation. A number of factors affect it, of which the main ones are:

■ the thickness and amount of the alveolar membrane,

■ the capillary blood volume,

■ the haemoglobin concentration (the test needs to be corrected for haemoglobin level).

Gas transfer is significantly reduced in more severe degrees of emphysema, because of the loss of alveolar tissue. (Gas transfer is also reduced in fibrosing alveolitis, allergic alveolitis and other causes of diffuse fibrosis.) In asthma, gas transfer is normal.

Static lung volumes (Figure 4.11)

Measurement of the total lung capacity (TLC) and residual volume (RV) using a body plethysmograph apparatus is occasionally used in hospital when assessing patients for lung surgery for COPD. In

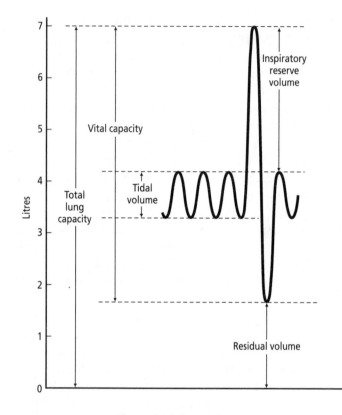

Figure 4.11 Lung volumes

emphysema, residual volume is greatly increased because of the volume of air trapped in enlarged air sacs and by airway collapse due to loss of the 'guy ropes' effect (see Chapter 2).

CT lung scans in inhalation and exhalation can also be used to measure lung volumes.

Further reading

BTS COPD Consortium (2000) *Spirometry in Practice*. British Thoracic Society, London [Available free via e-mail or fax (for contact details, see 'Useful addresses' section)]
Schermer TRJ, Folgering HTM, Bottema BJAM et al. (2000) The value of spirometry for primary care: asthma and COPD. *Primary Care Respiratory Journal* **9**: 51–5

5

Assessment

Main points

1 In most cases a diagnosis of COPD can be made on the basis of a thorough history and airflow obstruction on spirometry. Diagnostic reversibility testing is not necessary in all cases.

2 In cases of diagnostic doubt, the NICE guidelines suggest that an increase in the FEV_1 of 400ml or more in response to a bronchodilator or steroid reversibility test indicates asthma rather than COPD. Reversibility of less than this is not significant.

3 A negative response to a bronchodilator reversibility test does not mean that the patient will not benefit from long-term treatment with bronchodilators; therapeutic trials of several weeks' treatment should be undertaken. The response to a bronchodilator reversibility test does not indicate which bronchodilator is likely to give the most symptomatic benefit. Similarly, a steroid reversibility test cannot be used to determine which patients will benefit from inhaled steroids in the long term.

4 Patients with severe COPD who experience repeated exacerbations may benefit from long-term inhaled steroids even when they have no reversibility to a corticosteroid reversibility trial. (See 'Isolde' in Chapter 7.) Corticosteroid reversibility testing could be considered unnecessary in such patients, except to exclude asthma.

5 In patients presenting with severe disease, a referral for arterial blood gases is indicated, especially if the oxygen saturation is less than 92% and there are signs of cyanosis, raised jugular venous pressure, peripheral oedema or polycythaemia.

6 Other possible causes of the patient's symptoms must
   be considered and excluded. In the case of continued
   diagnostic uncertainty, the patient should be referred for
   a specialist opinion.

7 Formal assessments of disability and handicap should
   be performed as a baseline from which to assess the
   effectiveness of any treatment.

Making the diagnosis and establishing a baseline

Spirometry is essential to the diagnosis of COPD, and is discussed in
Chapter 4. It is crucial to the diagnosis of airway obstruction. A full
history (discussed in Chapter 3) is also needed. The history, signs
and symptoms are often sufficient to make a provisional diagnosis
of COPD. Sometimes it is difficult to differentiate between asthma
and COPD; Table 5.1 lists the main differentiating points.

Table 5.1 The main differentiating points between COPD and asthma

	COPD	*Asthma*
Current or or ex-smoker	Almost always	Possibly
Symptoms under the age of 45 years	Rarely	Often
Chronic productive cough	Common	Rare – may occur during exacerbations
Breathlessness	Persistent and progressive	Intermittent and variable
Night-time waking with cough and wheeze	Rare	Common
Diurnal or day-to-day variability of symptoms	Uncommon	Common

When the diagnosis is likely to be COPD, a therapeutic trial of
bronchodilators can be given and the patient reviewed after several
weeks of treatment to assess their response. COPD is unlikely if:

- The FEV_1 and the FEV_1/FVC ratio return to normal with drug therapy.

- The patient reports a dramatic improvement in their symptoms in response to inhaled bronchodilators.

When the history is not clear, reversibility testing with bronchodilators or steroids may help to clarify whether the patient has asthma or COPD.

Bronchodilator reversibility

The main objective of bronchodilator reversibility testing in COPD is to detect patients who have a substantial increase in the FEV_1, and are therefore suffering from asthma.

Reversibility testing was traditionally used to differentiate asthma from COPD and to help determine which bronchodilators were likely to be most effective. However, the evidence-based NICE guidelines have highlighted several problems with this approach:

- There is considerable variation in response from day to day in the same individual, and the results of reversibility tests performed on different occasions can be inconsistent and not reproducible.

- Previously suggested levels of positive response (15% and 200ml improvement in FEV_1) were arbitrary and were not based on evidence.

- Long-term symptomatic response to bronchodilators cannot be determined by the response to a dose of bronchodilator given during a reversibility test.

- Examination of inflammatory cells in bronchial biopsy and induced sputum samples revealed that asthma and COPD could generally be differentiated on the grounds of the clinical history. Reversibility tests were not able to differentiate between the two diseases.

Interpretation of acute bronchodilator response is difficult unless the improvement in FEV_1 is very large (greater than 400ml), in which case the patient is more likely to have asthma.

Where diagnostic doubt exists and bronchodilator reversibility tests are being considered, it is important to undertake them when the patient is clinically stable and free of infection.

Because small doses of bronchodilator will produce a response in fewer people, high doses of bronchodilator should be used in order not to miss a significant response. The most convenient way to deliver high-dose bronchodilators reliably is via a nebuliser, but repeated doses from a metered dose inhaler (MDI) through a spacer may be as effective. Suitable doses would be 400μg salbutamol or 80μg ipratropium, or the two combined.

- Record FEV_1 before and 15 minutes after giving 2.5–5mg nebulised salbutamol or 5–10mg nebulised terbutaline, or four puffs from an MDI via a spacer (one puff at a time).

- Record (preferably on a separate occasion) FEV_1 before and 30 minutes after 500μg nebulised ipratropium bromide, or four puffs from an MDI via a spacer

  or

- Record FEV_1 before and 30 minutes after a combination of salbutamol (or terbutaline) and ipratropium.

When the FEV_1 increases by 400ml or more, this will support a diagnosis of asthma. A response of less than this will support a diagnosis of COPD.

Even when there is no significant reversibility to bronchodilators on formal testing, patients with COPD still benefit from long-term bronchodilator therapy in terms of improved functional ability and well-being or decreased breathlessness. It is thought that, in the longer term, bronchodilators reduce air-trapping and over-inflation of the lungs, thus improving both respiratory muscle mechanics and exercise tolerance and breathlessness. Trials of several weeks of treatment with different drugs, different combinations of drugs and different doses are needed to establish which is the most effective treatment for each individual. The use of bronchodilators in COPD is discussed in Chapter 7.

The measures of outcome from therapeutic trials of bronchodilators in COPD are different from those used in the reversibility testing described above. Improvements in lung function cannot be anticipated and should not be sought. Improvements in functional ability and/or breathlessness are more significant. Methods of objectively measuring these rather subjective effects are discussed in detail later in this chapter.

The GOLD and NICE classifications of severity are shown in Table 5.2.

Table 5.2 GOLD and NICE classifications of severity

	GOLD classification	NICE classification
Mild disease	FEV_1 >80% predicted but FEV_1/FVC <70% (stage I)	FEV_1 50–80% predicted
Moderate disease	FEV_1 30–80% predicted (stage IIA) 50–80% predicted + respiratory or right heart failure (stage IIB)	FEV_1 30–49% predicted
Severe disease	FEV_1 <30% predicted or FEV_1 <50% predicted + chronic respiratory or right heart failure	FEV_1 < 30% predicted

The prognosis is directly related to the FEV_1 and inversely related to the patient's age. The post-bronchodilator value correlates better with survival than the pre-bronchodilator value:

- Aged under 60 and FEV_1 above 50% predicted — 90% 3-year survival
- Aged over 60 and FEV_1 above 50% predicted — 80% 3-year survival
- Aged over 60 and FEV_1 40–49% predicted — 75% 3-year survival

Corticosteroid reversibility

A positive response to an oral steroid trial is most likely in patients who have achieved significant reversibility in bronchodilator reversibility tests. Steroid reversibility helps identify people with asthma. It is not a method of identifying which COPD patients need long-term inhaled steroids. The use of inhaled steroids in COPD is discussed in Chapter 7 and 12.

As with bronchodilator reversibility tests, corticosteroid reversibility testing should be done during a period of clinical stability.

The NICE guidelines recommend that prednisolone 30mg is given daily for two weeks. The GOLD guidelines suggest that a trial of between six weeks and three months on high-dose inhaled steroids (1000µg of beclometasone per day or an equivalent dose of an alternative inhaled steroid) may be a safer and more reliable method. Spirometry is recorded before and immediately at the end of the trial. The response should be measured in terms of the *post-bronchodilator* FEV_1. In other words, the FEV_1 is measured after administering an adequate dose of bronchodilator both at the start and at the end of the trial. An improvement of 400ml or more in the FEV_1 indicates that the patient has asthma rather than COPD, and they will require long-term inhaled steroids. Data from the Isolde trial have demonstrated that improvements of less than this are not significant.

The usefulness of long-term inhaled steroids in COPD has been the subject of intensive research and their role has become clearer. This is discussed in detail in Chapters 7 and 12.

Excluding alternative and coexisting pathologies

Lung cancer is an important differential diagnosis to consider. The incidence of lung cancer is high among patients with COPD. Indeed, there is some evidence that smokers who have COPD have a higher risk of developing lung cancer than smokers who are not susceptible to COPD. It is therefore important to maintain a high index of suspicion of lung cancer in patients with COPD. Any middle-aged or older smoker presenting with respiratory symptoms should have a chest x-ray to exclude this. By the time symptoms arise most, though not all, lung cancers are visible on chest x-ray.

If the chest x-ray reveals 'emphysematous changes' or 'hyper-inflation', this will add weight to a diagnosis of COPD, although hyperinflation may also be a feature of chronic asthma. Emphysema may be assessed by computed tomography (CT) – see Figure 5.1. CT can also be used in the diagnosis of bronchiectasis, a condition found in 29% of COPD patients with persistent cough and sputum as an accompanying disease process.

A chest x-ray may show bullous emphysema, which might be

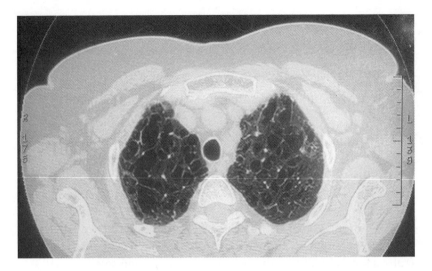

Figure 5.1 A CT scan, showing emphysema

treated surgically. It may reveal cardiac enlargement and pulmonary oedema, prompting cardiac investigation.

The chest x-ray need not be repeated routinely, but an unexplained change in symptoms should be regarded with suspicion. Often the change in symptoms is reported by the patient's carer and is rather ill-defined and vague: 'He just hasn't been the same recently'. Such a history, failure of a chest infection to resolve or haemoptysis merits a repeat chest x-ray to exclude a tumour.

An electrocardiogram will help in the differential diagnosis of cardiac breathlessness, provided it is correctly interpreted. In some areas, there is open access to echocardiography. A review of the patient's current medication may also lend weight to a diagnosis of cardiac breathlessness or reveal the use of beta-blockade which may have precipitated asthma.

A full blood count should be taken to exclude anaemia as a cause of breathlessness. It will also reveal polycythaemia in the chronically hypoxic patient. A referral for arterial blood gases is indicated if polycythaemia is present.

The GOLD guidelines recommend referral for arterial blood gases in all patients with an FEV_1 less than 40% predicted. The NICE guidelines recommend referral for patients with severe disease (FEV_1<30% predicted) and suggest that referral be considered in patients with less severe disease (FEV_1<50% predicted) if they have one or more of:

- cyanosis,

- peripheral oedema,

- raised jugular venous pressure,

- oxygen saturation less than 92%, when clinically stable.

It should be remembered that cyanosis is an unreliable clinical sign and may not become apparent until the oxygen saturation is down to 85% or less. NICE recommends that pulse oximeters should be available in all settings to allow accurate and objective assessment of patients. If the oxygen saturation is over 92%, arterial blood gases may not be necessary at that time.

Oximeters, whilst useful for detecting hypoxia, are unable to detect hypercapnia (raised levels of CO_2). Hypoxia and hypercapnia (raised levels of CO_2 in the blood) are common in severe COPD.

Diseases that cause pulmonary fibrosis (e.g. fibrosing alveolitis) may present as breathlessness on exertion and may be confused with COPD. However, the spirometry will not reveal obstruction. The FEV_1/FVC ratio will be normal or high but the lung volumes, the FEV_1 and the FVC will be low. Patients with this pattern of restricted spirometry require assessment by a respiratory physician and are generally beyond the scope of primary care management.

Severe obstructive sleep apnoea (OSA) can present as cor pulmonale. The upper airway obstructs during sleep, producing repeated apnoea sufficient to cause a significant drop in oxygen saturation levels and to rouse the sufferer repeatedly. Patients have a history of 'heroic' snoring and they complain of daytime somnolence. They may have a poor driving accident record because they fall asleep at the wheel. OSA is more common in men than women, and sufferers are often obese, with a collar size of 17 inches or more. Although OSA is an upper respiratory problem and is not related to COPD, it may coexist with it, particularly in patients who are overweight or Cushingoid due to long-term use of oral steroids.

Disability and handicap

Once it has been established that the patient has irreversible airflow obstruction and alternative diagnoses have been excluded, it is important to measure the impact of the disease on the patient's everyday life: the level of disability and handicap. These considerations are frequently overlooked, but it is these effects that are most important to the patient and are the areas that treatment of COPD aims to improve.

Because airways obstruction is largely fixed, big improvements in lung function are not attainable but improvements in disability and handicap are. For the patient such outcomes are far more important than, for example, an improvement of 100ml in the FEV_1, because they equate more with their ability to carry on their everyday lives. You will need a baseline level of disability and handicap from which to assess accurately the effectiveness of any intervention.

Assessing breathlessness

'Breathlessness' is a subjective term, but it is important to quantify this feature because improvement in breathlessness is one of the most important ways of seeing whether treatment is working. There are several scales for assessing it objectively.

The MRC dyspnoea scale (Table 5.3) allows patients to rate their breathlessness according to the activity that induces it. It is graded from 0 to 5.

Whilst the MRC scale is helpful and easy to use, it is relatively insensitive to change and may be more valuable as a baseline assessment or monitoring tool rather than a means of measuring the effect of a treatment.

Table 5.3 MRC dyspnoea scale

Grade	Degree of breathlessness related to activities
0	Not troubled by breathlessness except on strenuous exercise
1	Short of breath when hurrying or walking up a slight hill
2	Walks slower than contemporaries on the level because of breathlessness, or has to stop for breath when walking at own pace
3	Stops for breath after walking about 100m or after a few minutes on the level
4	Too breathless to leave the house, or breathless when dressing or undressing
5	Breathless at rest

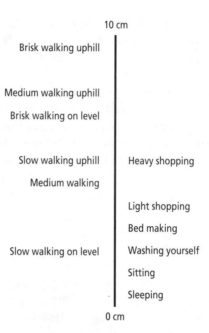

Figure 5.2 The 'oxygen cost' diagram

The oxygen cost diagram is more sensitive to change than the MRC scale; it allows the patient to place a mark on a 10cm line, beyond which they become breathless (Figure 5.2). The ability score is the distance in centimetres from the zero point.

Table 5.4 The Borg scale

0	Nothing at all
0.5	Very, very slight (just noticeable)
1	Very slight
2	Slight (light)
3	Moderate
4	Somewhat severe
5	Severe (heavy)
6	
7	Very severe
8	
9	
10	Very, very severe (almost maximal)
	Maximal

Other scales allow patients to grade their breathlessness according to the intensity of the sensation. The Borg scale (Table 5.4) is useful for measuring short-term changes in the intensity of the breathlessness during a particular task. It is both sensitive and reproducible.

A simple visual analogue scale is another method of allowing patients to rate the intensity of their breathlessness. As with the oxygen cost diagram, a 10cm line is drawn on a page and the patient then marks on the line how intense their breathlessness is, from 0cm (nothing at all) to 10cm (intensely breathless). The score is the distance along the line that the patient has marked.

Assessing walking distance

A six-minute walking test and a shuttle walking test are also methods of objectively measuring disability. The six-minute walk measures the distance a patient can walk in six minutes, indoors, on the flat. The patient does a practice walk first, to give them confidence, and measurements are taken on the second walk. The patient is actively encouraged throughout, and stops for rest are allowed. In a shuttle test the patient performs a paced walk between two points 10 metres apart (a shuttle). The pace of the walk is increased at regular intervals, dictated by 'beeps' on a tape recording, until the patient is forced to stop because of breathlessness. The number of completed shuttles is then recorded.

If neither the six-minute walk nor the shuttle walking test is feasible in the practice, you should ask the patient how far they are able to walk; comparisons between walking distance before and after any intervention can still be useful. Asking how many lamp posts the patient can walk past before they get breathless, before and after a given intervention, may be a practical way to assess walking distance objectively in a primary care setting.

If no objective measurements of disability or walking distance have been taken, the effect of an intervention can be assessed by asking:

■ Has your treatment made a difference to you?

■ Is your breathing easier in any way?

■ Can you do some things now that you couldn't do before, or the same things but faster?

- Can you do the same things as before but are now less breathless when you do them?

- Has your sleep improved?

Assessing the impact of the disease on daily activities

The progressively disabling nature of COPD means that it will eventually affect a patient's ability to carry out their normal, every-day activities. The London Chest Activities of Daily Living (LCADL) questionnaire aims to assess this aspect of the impact of COPD. It is a 15-item questionnaire for the patient to complete. It is quick and simple to do. However, it is suitable only for patients with severe disease.

Impact of the disease on psychosocial functioning

Increasing disability and breathlessness on exertion eventually affect all areas of the patient's psychological, sexual and social functioning. An individual's perception of their health status is closely associated with their personality and the amount of social support they have; those with supportive families do better than those who live alone. Some patients with relatively good lung function may be significantly disabled, have given up work and be isolated and depressed, whereas others with appalling lung function may continue to work and remain active and cheerful.

Attacks of breathlessness frequently produce feelings of fear and panic. Episodes in public can cause anxiety and embarrassment, and the wish to avoid such feelings may well sow the seeds of social isolation. Depression is common, significantly affecting an individual's ability to cope with the disease and lessening the effectiveness of any therapeutic intervention. Treating coexisting depression can have a very significant beneficial effect on the patient's health status and overall quality of life.

Loss of independence frequently causes feelings of anger, frustration or resentment, often manifested as impatience with the person closest to the patient. Such feelings result in loss of self-esteem and may cause self-destructive behaviour, such as a refusal to stop smoking. The way that patients often cope with these very negative feelings is to withdraw physically and emotionally. Many COPD patients live in an 'emotional straitjacket' (see Chapter 8).

Assessing health status

Assessing health status in COPD, like measuring breathlessness and disability, is important because it too may be improved.

There are several questionnaires available for the measurement of health status, mostly used in hospital rehabilitation programmes and research. The Chronic Respiratory Disease Index Questionnaire is very sensitive to change, but is also the most cumbersome and time consuming to use, and requires training to administer properly. It was developed as a research tool, requires training to administer and is really not practical for everyday use. To overcome some of these problems, a shorter version of this questionnaire, which the patient fills in, has recently been developed and validated. The St George's Respiratory Questionnaire, a 'self-fill' questionnaire, is more practical and is also available in a shortened version, the AQ20. Another 'self-fill' questionnaire is the Breathing Problems Questionnaire. This is user-friendly and is also available in a short version.

In practice, many of these questionnaires are too cumbersome and time consuming. Their advantages and disadvantages are summarised in Table 5.5. Such formal questionnaires are most useful in the setting of a formal rehabilitation programme. In general practice, a simple enquiry about the two or three most distressing daily activities may suffice. Include questions about the patient's overall feelings of fatigue and about their emotional state. Depression may manifest itself as panic, anxiety or feelings of helplessness and hopelessness.

The degree of control that a patient feels may be assessed by asking such questions as:

- 'How confident do you feel about dealing with your illness?'

- 'Do you feel upset or frightened by your attacks of breathlessness?'

- 'Do you feel in control of your breathlessness?'

- 'Do you feel tired?'

- 'Do you ever feel down?'

Table 5.5 Health status questionnaires compared

Measure	Description	Advantages	Disadvantages
St George's Respiratory Questionnaire (SGRQ)	76 items Patient self-completes Assesses symptoms, activity, impact on daily life One total score Weighted scoring system	Reproducible and sensitive Well established and validated in many countries 'Gold standard' measure	Time consuming to complete Complicated to to score Some patients have difficulty understanding the questions
AQ20	20 items Patient self-completes Yes/No answers only	Takes 2 minutes to complete and score Repeatable and sensitive	Less sensitive for patients with mild health status impairment
Chronic Respiratory Questionnaire (CRQ)	20 items Both self-fill and interviewer-administered versions Four components (dyspnoea, fatigue, emotional functioning, mastery) Individualised by patient Weighted scoring system	Reproducible and sensitive Well studied	Time consuming to complete and score Scoring system complicated

Summary

Middle-aged or older patients with respiratory symptoms, particularly those with a significant smoking history, pose a challenge to the health professional. There may have been a tendency to class all breathless smokers as suffering from COPD but it is extremely important not to become blinkered. Asthma can occur at any age, regardless of smoking status. Smokers are at risk of many other smoking-related diseases, such as ischaemic heart disease or lung cancer, and they may have other lung disease or coexisting pathologies that make assessment difficult.

It is therefore extremely important that history taking is thorough and comprehensive and that alternative diagnosis is ruled out. It is also vital that patients are reviewed to assess their response to treatment and, when there is any degree of diagnostic uncertainty, further tests carried out to confirm or refute a diagnosis of COPD. Failure to assess patients properly may lead to misdiagnosis and inappropriate treatment. All patients deserve a thorough assessment to make sure that other pathologies are not missed and that appropriate treatment is given and its effectiveness properly assessed.

Further reading

Assessment of impairment

BRITISH THORACIC SOCIETY (1997) BTS guidelines for the management of chronic obstructive pulmonary disease. *Thorax* **52** (Suppl 5): S1–S28

BURROWS B (1991) Predictors of cause and prognosis of obstructive lung disease. *European Respiratory Review* **1**: 340–5

CALLAHAN CM, CITTUS RS, KATZ BP (1991) Oral corticosteroid therapy for patients with stable chronic obstructive pulmonary disease: a meta-analysis. *Annals of Internal Medicine* **114**: 216–23

ROBERTS CM, BUGLER JR, MELCHOR R et al. (1993) Value of pulse oximetry for long-term oxygen requirement. *European Respiratory Journal* **6**: 559–62

Assessment of disability

BORG G (1982) Psychophysical basis of perceived exertion. *Medicine and Science in Sports and Exercise* **14**: 377–81

GARROD R, BESTALL JC, PAUL EA et al. (2000) Development and validation of a standardized measure of activity of daily living in patients with severe COPD: the London Chest Activity of Daily Living Scale (LCADL). *Respiratory Medicine* **94**: 589–96

McGAVIN CR, ARTVINLI M, NAOE H (1978) Dyspnoea, disability and distance walked: a comparison of estimates of exercise performance in respiratory disease. *British Medical Journal* **2**: 241–3

NOSEDA A, CARPEIAUX JP, SCHMERBER J (1992) Dyspnoea assessed by visual analogue scale in patients with obstructive lung disease during progressive and high intensity exercise. *Thorax* **47**: 363–8

SINGH SJ, MORGAN MDL, SCOTT SC et al. (1992) The development of the shuttle walking test of disability in patients with chronic airways obstruction. *Thorax* **47**: 1019–24

WILLIAMS SJ, BURY MR (1989) Impairment, disability and handicap in chronic respiratory illness. *Social Science and Medicine* **29** (5): 609–16

Assessment of handicap

DUDLEY DL, GLASER EM, JORGENSON BN et al. (1980) Psychosocial concomitants to rehabilitation in chronic obstructive pulmonary disease. *Chest* **77** (3): 413–20

GUYATT GH, BERMAN LB, TOWNSEND M et al. (1987) A measure of quality of life for clinical trials in chronic lung disease. *Thorax* **42**: 773–8

HYLAND ME, BOTT J, SING S, KENYON CAP (1994) Domains, constructs and the development of the breathing problems questionnaire. *Quality of Life Research* **3**: 245–56

JONES PW, QUIRK FH, BAVEYSTOCK CM et al. (1992) A self-complete measure for chronic airflow limitation: the St George's questionnaire. *American Review of Respiratory Disease* **147**: 832–8

O'BRIEN C, GUEST PJ, HILL SL, STOCKLEY RA (2000) Physiological and radiological characterisation of patients diagnosed with chronic obstructive pulmonary disease in primary care. *Thorax* **55**: 635–42

Addresses for questionnaires

Chronic Respiratory Disease Index Questionnaires
Peggy Austin and Dr Holger Schünemann
Room 2C12
McMaster University Health Sciences Centre
Hamilton, Ontario L8N 3Z5
CANADA
Email: austinp@mcmaster.ca or schuneh@mcmaster.ca

St George's Respiratory Questionnaire
Professor Paul Jones
Division of Physiological Medicine
St George's Hospital Medical School
Cranmer Terrace
London SW17 0RE

Breathing Problems Questionnaire
Professor Michael Hyland
Department of Psychology
University of Plymouth
Plymouth
Devon PL4 8AA

London Chest Activities of Daily Living
R Garrod
Academic Respiratory Department
St Bartholomew's and Royal London School of Medicine
and Dentistry
Turner Street
London E1 2AD

6 Smoking cessation

Main points

1 Stopping smoking is the only intervention that significantly affects the natural history of COPD.

2 Brief advice from health professionals can be effective in persuading people to stop smoking.

3 The use of nicotine replacement therapy (NRT) can double long-term quit rates.

4 Matching patient to product may be helpful. Gum, inhalator, nasal spray or sublingual tablets may be most helpful for the heavily addicted smoker.

5 Bupropion, a non-nicotine oral treatment, can at least double long-term/one-year smoking-cessation rates.

6 The National Institute for Clinical Excellence have endorsed the use of bupropion and NRT in smokers who are ready to stop.

7 Support and follow-up of patients, particularly through the critical first two to three weeks, may also increase quit rates.

Stopping smoking is the single most important intervention in COPD and the only thing that significantly alters the natural history of the disease. It is of primary importance at every stage and must be encouraged actively and continuously. In mild COPD it may be the only treatment needed and may prevent the patient ever developing severe, disabling and life-threatening illness.

Unfortunately, persuading patients to stop smoking is often difficult, and failure can be demoralising and disheartening for patient and health professional alike. Most ex-smokers have made several serious attempts to stop before they eventually succeed. A 10% success rate is good!

Why do people smoke?

The reasons why people start smoking and continue to smoke in the face of mounting evidence of its harmful effects are complex. Currently 28% of adult males and 26% of adult females are smokers and 26% of the population are ex-smokers. Smoking rates are highest among lower socio-economic groups. Rising tobacco taxation and increasing evidence of the harmful effects of smoking have little effect on people in these groups. Perversely, those who can least afford it – the economically deprived – are those who tend to smoke, continue to smoke and smoke most!

Most smokers start in adolescence, when it may be seen as a 'rite of passage' to adulthood. There may be considerable and irresistible peer group pressure to smoke. Smoking may be one of those 'risk-taking' or rebellious behaviours that are a normal part of growing up. Unfortunately, a third of the adolescents who start will become life-long smokers, and 450 children start smoking every day. Health education messages about the long-term effects of smoking have little effect. In the UK about 300 adults die of a smoking-related disease every day, so the tobacco industry needs to recruit new smokers to replace them!

Nicotine is highly addictive and smokers are adept at adjusting their smoking to satisfy their need for nicotine without taking in so much that they suffer side-effects. It is also a powerful neural stimulant, acting on the pleasure centres of the brain. Stimulation is followed by rebound depression and the addicted smoker then feels the need for another cigarette. The biochemistry of a nicotine-addicted brain is different from that in a 'normal' brain.

- The cigarette is a highly efficient nicotine-delivery system. Nicotine is absorbed very rapidly across the lungs and reaches the brain quicker than if it were injected intravenously.

- If the number of cigarettes smoked a day is reduced, the smoker will take longer and deeper puffs to get the same amount of nicotine.

- Reducing the number smoked or switching to a lower tar cigarette is seldom successful as a quitting strategy.

■ Cigarette smokers who switch to cigars are likely to inhale the cigar smoke and get an even higher tar load into the lungs than with cigarettes.

Nicotine, although addictive, is a relatively harmless drug. It is the other constituents of tobacco that cause damage. Cigarette smoke contains upwards of 4000 different chemicals, 600 of which are known carcinogens. Perrier water was withdrawn from sale when it was found to contain 4.7μg per litre of benzene, a known carcinogen. A single cigarette delivers 190μg of benzene!

Addiction to nicotine is the main reason why smokers find it hard to stop, but there are other factors. Each cigarette is 'puffed' about 10–12 times, and 20 cigarettes a day is associated with 200–250 hand-to-mouth movements every day: 91,250 movements a year. A powerful habit! Smoking becomes associated with pleasurable everyday activities: having a cup of coffee, relaxing after a meal, watching the television etc. It may be associated with pleasurable memories and social activities. When smokers try to quit they not only have to cope with withdrawal of an addictive drug but also with the loss of an 'old friend' that might have been part of their lives for many years. Fear of failure may be another powerful reason why a smoker does not make any move to stop. Physical addiction and habit together serve to make smoking a very difficult habit to break.

How can smokers stop smoking?

In order to stop, the smoker has to *want* to stop. This sounds painfully obvious but the path from 'contented smoker' to serious 'quitter' is tortuous and one where advice from you can have a considerable influence. Some health professionals find it difficult to engage with smokers about their behaviour, fearing that advice to give up may damage their relationship with that patient and 'scare them off'. Raising the subject needs to done sensitively and in a non-threatening manner. The use of 'open' questions that encourage the smoker to talk about their habit and how they feel about stopping can be a helpful way of beginning to address the issue. Nearly 70% of smokers, when asked, say they would like to stop, so constructive advice, support and encouragement might help them to move from a period of contemplation to doing something serious about quitting. Tagging the medical records and bringing up the subject of smoking in a non-threatening way at every attendance can be highly effective and may prompt a 'contented smoker' to contemplate stopping, or a smoker who is contemplating stopping to making a serious attempt to stop. Showing concern, acknowledging the difficulties of quitting and offering practical advice and support are perhaps most helpful. A censorious approach is likely to produce only resistance, and a lecture about the harmful effects of smoking is likely to be counter-productive. Smokers know that their habit is harmful! It is more effective to ask what they think would be the benefits of stopping and to relate and reinforce those benefits in relation to their own health. For a smoker with COPD this is relatively easy. Relating their own lung function to what it would be in a healthy non-smoker (see Figure 2.2) could be a powerful incentive to take a serious step to becoming an ex-smoker. Positive encouragement that stopping smoking is a really effective and important step that they can take to help themselves, together with reassurance that you will be there to help, may be the best approach.

A dramatic event (e.g. a myocardial infarction) that makes a patient anxious about their health is often a trigger to action. Unfortunately, slowly progressive breathlessness seldom produces the same trigger, but a recent unpleasant chest infection or exacerbation of COPD might. Targeting patients when they are most susceptible to advice may increase success rates.

Once a patient has decided to make a serious attempt to stop smoking, practical advice on how to cope and support through the first critical three months of stopping are most beneficial. 'Quit smoking' groups are available in some areas for people who feel they would benefit from a support group. Alternatively, follow-up appointments at the surgery or health centre at one week, three weeks, two months and three months after stopping to offer support and encouragement may be helpful. If your resources are strained, the most important period to concentrate on is the first month. It may take several serious attempts before a smoker makes the final transition to ex-smoker. In the event of relapse, it is important not to condemn but rather to support and encourage the patient to try to identify why they have failed, develop a strategy for avoiding failure in the future and to make another serious attempt. As Mark Twain famously remarked:

'Stopping smoking is easy. I've done it hundreds of times.'

Nicotine replacement therapy

For some smokers, withdrawal symptoms such as irritability, nervousness and cravings may cause relapse and unwillingness to make another attempt to quit. Nicotine replacement therapy (NRT) can be very effective; large, placebo-controlled trials have shown that it can approximately double quit rates at one year. It is available in six forms:

- chewing gum,

- transdermal patch,

- inhalator,

- nasal spray,

- sublingual tablet,

- lozenge.

Figure 6.1 shows the different blood nicotine levels with the different types. All forms of NRT are available both 'over the counter' at pharmacists and on prescription in the UK.

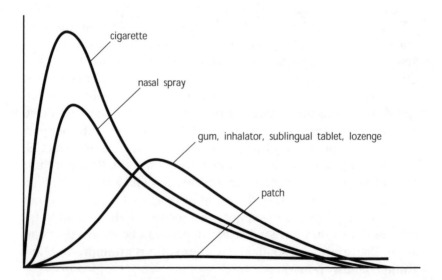

Figure 6.1 Blood nicotine levels with different types of nicotine replacement therapy

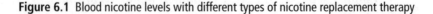

Nicotine gum

This is the oldest form of NRT and is available in two strengths (2mg and 4mg) and a variety of flavours. The gum should be chewed until it starts to produce a flavour and then 'parked' between the cheek and the gum. If it is chewed continuously, it tastes unpleasant. When the desire to smoke is felt again, the gum is chewed and parked again. Each piece of gum lasts about 20 minutes and up to 16 pieces can be chewed in 24 hours. Nicotine is absorbed from the lining of the mouth, the buccal mucosa, and produces a peak in venous nicotine levels similar in shape but less than that achieved by smoking. It is suitable for the highly addicted smoker because it is used on demand.

Nasal spray

The peaks in nicotine level that can be achieved with a nasal spray are higher than can be obtained with the gum but still considerably lower than those achieved with cigarettes. The nicotine is absorbed from the nasal mucosa. It should not be sniffed up the nose but sprayed onto the mucosa when the desire to smoke is felt. Up to 64 'puffs' a day can be used. This form of NRT most closely resembles the effects of smoking and is most suitable for the very heavily addicted smoker. Until recently it was available only on a private prescription, but has now, like all the other forms of NRT, become available 'over the counter' and on NHS prescription.

Nicotine inhalator

The inhalator produces peaks in nicotine levels similar to those from nicotine gum. The inhalator contains a mentholated plug impregnated with nicotine, and is sucked when the desire to smoke is felt and until that desire goes away. Nicotine is absorbed from the buccal mucosa. Each plug lasts for about 20 minutes.

Nicotine patches

Transdermal patches are easy to use. They are of two types (16 hour or 24 hour), and come in several strengths. Patches do not produce peaks in nicotine levels to mimic the effect of smoking but, rather, provide a steady background level. The rationale behind the

24-hour patch is to prevent the strong urge to smoke that many smokers feel first thing in the morning, caused by an overnight fall in nicotine levels. They may, however, produce sleep disturbance or nightmares, and the adhesive in the patches can cause local skin irritation.

Sublingual tablets

When the desire to smoke is felt, a tablet is dissolved under the tongue. The peak in nicotine level obtained is similar to that achieved with gum or the inhalator, and, because they too are used on demand, sublingual tablets are suitable for heavily addicted smokers. Unlike the other forms of NRT, these tablets are licensed for use during pregnancy, if the woman is unable to stop smoking without using NRT.

Lozenges

Lozenges are also used on demand and are suitable for the heavily addicted smoker. They produce peaks in nicotine levels similar to those achieved with sublingual tablets, inhalator and gum. One or two lozenges can be sucked per hour, when the urge to smoke is felt.

The principle of NRT is to replace the nicotine a smoker takes in, although at considerably lower levels, thus reducing withdrawal symptoms and allowing the smoker to concentrate on changing the habits of smoking. When the habit is broken, the amount of nicotine can be reduced over a period and the NRT withdrawn. It is important that the smoker understands at the outset that it is not intended to replace cigarettes and will not be a substitute for will power. A considerable amount of nicotine will be given up from day one. In order for NRT to work, the smoker has to be motivated to stop! It is not suitable for the genuinely light or social smoker, because it may provide more nicotine than they are accustomed to and produce toxic side-effects.

To maximise success with NRT it may help if you match the smoker to the product and ensure that the smoker's expectations of the effects of NRT are realistic. Instruction in how to chew the gum or use the inhalator may prevent problems with incorrect use. Failure with NRT is often due to:

Staffordshire University
School of Health
Royal Shrewsbury Hospital (North)

- stopping therapy too soon,

- not using high enough doses because of fears about side-effects,

- concurrent smoking – a potentially dangerous practice.

The list of possible side-effects on the side of a packet of NRT can be daunting. Fear of side-effects may also be used as an excuse not to attempt to stop smoking, and some smokers are concerned about becoming addicted to the NRT! This is in fact a rare occurrence, so you can reassure patients that this is unlikely.

It is important that patients understand that the side-effects of NRT are the same as the side-effects of smoking but that the risks of using it are considerably less than those of continuing to smoke. Except for the sublingual tablets (see earlier), however, NRT should *not* be used by pregnant or breast-feeding women because of the lack of research into its teratogenicity. It is also advised that NRT not be used:

- within three months of a myocardial infarction,

- within three months of a cerebrovascular accident,

- by people with active peptic ulceration,

although for these patients the risks of continuing to smoke are probably considerably higher.

Transdermal patches should not be used by patients with extensive skin disease; the other types of NRT – chewing gum, nasal spray, inhalator, sublingual tablets or lozenges – should be used instead.

Generally, NRT should be taken for 12 weeks with a two- to four-week period at the end of the course when the dose is reduced. The benefits of using NRT and stopping smoking massively outweigh the risks of continuing to smoke, and helping patients to come to grips with the reality of the risks may be helpful.

Specialist centres will sometimes recommend the use of two different forms of NRT concurrently – patches and gum, for example – if the smoker is very heavily dependent and unable to stop. However, this is outside the normal licence for NRT and specialist care may be needed for such 'problem' smokers.

Bupropion

Bupropion was initially developed as an antidepressant. It works directly on the addiction pathways in the brain and helps to prevent cravings for nicotine rather than replacing one nicotine delivery system with another. It can be very effective, although, like NRT, it is not a replacement for will power and the smoker has to be motivated to stop. Several large, placebo-controlled studies have demonstrated its effectiveness. It has produced a sustained quit rate of up to 30% when combined with counselling and support. One study has shown it to be effective in helping COPD patients to quit. Over all, it has had better quit rates than other smoking-cessation methods, and has been endorsed by the National Institute for Clinical Excellence (NICE) as a cost-effective therapy.

An agreed 'quit date' is set at about 10–17 days into the course of treatment and the smoker can continue to smoke until then. One bupropion 150mg tablet a day is taken for six days then one twice daily, at least eight hours apart, for the remainder of the two-month course. The smoker stops smoking on the quit date but continues taking bupropion for a full eight weeks. The tablets can then be stopped abruptly. If the smoker has failed to stop after one month of treatment, they are unlikely to succeed and consideration should be given to stopping treatment after one month. A further course at a later date, when the reasons for failure have been addressed, may be successful. A combination of bupropion and NRT patches has been given with good effect in some specialist centres.

Bupropion is generally well tolerated. Side-effects such as insomnia, dry mouth, nausea, agitation or a generalised rash are experienced by a few smokers but these are usually mild and usually disappear once treatment is stopped.

There are some contraindications to its use, and prescribers and those who advise smokers must be fully conversant with them. They are:

- current or past seizures,
- current or past eating disorder (e.g. bulimia or anorexia nervosa),
- history of bipolar disorder (e.g. manic–depressive psychosis),
- severe hepatic cirrhosis,

■ brain tumour,

■ undergoing withdrawal from alcohol or benzodiazepines.

The prescribing information for bupropion also counsels caution when using this drug in smokers with any predisposing risk factors for seizure, such as concurrent use of other antidepressants, antipsychotics or theophyllines. Careful enquiry should therefore be made about concurrent drug use – including over-the-counter therapies such as St John's wort – and previous medical history.

When bupropion was first introduced in the UK there were a few, highly publicised, deaths associated with its use. However, that there was a causal link between the use of bupropion and these deaths is disputed. Most of the patients who died had underlying smoking-related conditions and some were not taking the drug at the time of their death. Others had contraindications to the use of bupropion that had not been reported to the prescriber.

It must be borne in mind, however, that every day in the UK there are at least 300 deaths that can be directly attributed to smoking. One in every two life-long smokers will die as a consequence of their habit; very poor odds! Nicotine addiction is difficult to overcome and bupropion is a very useful weapon in the fight against the addiction. The risks of continuing to smoke far outweigh the risks of using bupropion, provided it is given to carefully selected people. World wide, this therapy has helped millions of smokers to stop!

Helping patients to stop smoking

Helping patients to stop smoking can be the most rewarding and the most frustrating of tasks. However, it is the single most important thing you can do to improve the health of your patient. You must ask the smoker about their smoking habits and offer support and advice at every attendance. It is tempting sometimes not to bother to raise the subject because you know that you have discussed smoking cessation with that patient many times and your advice hasn't been heeded. But this may be the one time when you may make a difference! The following hints may be helpful.

Practical hints for health professionals

- Raise the subject of smoking cessation in a non-threatening way.

- Assess motivation to quit by asking open questions such as 'How do you feel about stopping smoking?'

- Show concern and offer appropriate advice/leaflets to the 'contented' smoker.

- Talking about the 'risks' of smoking can be counter-productive. Instead, ask the smoker what they see as the benefits of stopping.

- Make a record of a smoker's reasons for wanting to stop so that you can refer back to it with them.

- Acknowledge that stopping can be difficult, and offer constructive support and advice.

- Make a record of what you have advised, so that you do not repeat yourself and can recap and move forward next time.

- Record what the smoker has said to you. You can use it as a starting point when you next meet!

- Discuss the benefits of nicotine replacement therapy or bupropion. Help smokers to select and use their chosen form of treatment correctly.

- Follow up smokers during their attempt to quit.

- If they don't succeed, encourage them to try again.

The key recommendations for health professionals are:

- **Ask** about the smoking status of patients at every opportunity.

- **Advise** all smokers to stop.

- **Assist** those interested in doing so.

- **Arrange** follow-up.

- **Refer** to specialist cessation services if necessary.

■ **Recommend NRT (or bupropion)** to smokers who want to stop, and provide accurate advice about these treatments.

Practical hints for patients

1 *Set a 'quit' date.*
Stopping smoking is something you need to plan. It is seldom successful if it is undertaken on the spur of the moment, and gently cutting back is not effective. The best way to stop is just to stop.

Before quitting it may be helpful to keep a smoking diary so that danger times can be highlighted and strategies formulated for avoiding them.

Family and friends need to be informed so that they don't put temptation in your way.

2 *If possible, quit with a friend.*
Success rates are much higher when people have support and reinforcement available.

You may find Quit (the smoking quitlines) helpful. The telephone numbers are:

England: 0800 00 22 00
Northern Ireland: 02890 663 281
Scotland: 0800 84 84 84
Wales: 0800 169 0169 (national number)

3 *Consider using nicotine replacement therapy or bupropion (Zyban).*
They are not a replacement for your will power but can help you cope with cravings and can double your chances of success. Discuss this with your doctor or nurse.

The pharmaceutical companies that make bupropion and nicotine replacement products include in the packs of treatment 'helpline' information and leaflets to help you quit successfully. Some also provide a special service that you can register with for additional support during your quit attempt.

4 *On 'quit day' get rid of all cigarettes, lighters and ash trays.*

5 *Cash, not ash.*
Put aside the money you would have spent on smoking and reward yourself after a week or a fortnight.

6 *Avoid replacing cigarettes with extra cups of coffee or tea.*
Caffeine levels will be increased when you stop smoking and unpleasant side-effects (e.g. headaches) may occur. It is better to drink plenty of water or fruit juice.

7 *Cravings are short lived.*
Try to avoid situations where you would normally smoke. For example, instead of sitting down with a cup of coffee after a meal, get up and do something different. It may be advisable to stay away from the pub or from friends who smoke for the critical first two or three weeks. Alcohol may also weaken your power to resist a cigarette. Work out ways to distract yourself when cravings occur, to occupy you until they pass.

8 *Keep a 'nibble box' of raw carrots, celery or some other non-fattening food.*
Weight gain is common (average weight gain is about 4 kilograms). Don't try to diet and quit smoking at the same time, but do try to avoid sucking sweets and eating fattening foods to overcome your craving for cigarettes. As you begin to feel fitter, try taking up some form of exercise. This will help to keep your weight down and improve your general fitness. Exercising can also distract you from your cravings.

9 *Take it one day at a time.*
Tell yourself 'Today, I am not going to have a cigarette.'

10 *If you don't succeed this time – try again!*
Work out why you have failed and then try again. Learn from your mistakes.

Further reading

BRITISH THORACIC SOCIETY (1998) Smoking cessation guidelines and their cost effectiveness. *Thorax* **53** (Suppl 5): S1–38

NATIONAL ASTHMA AND RESPIRATORY TRAINING CENTRE (1999) *Simply Stop Smoking*. Direct Publishing Solutions, Cookham, Berks

NATIONAL INSTITUTE FOR CLINICAL EXCELLENCE (2002) *Guidance on the use of nicotine replacement therapy and bupropion for smoking cessation*. Technology Appraisal Guidance no. 39. NICE, London

PROCHASKA JO, DiCLEMENTE CC (1986) Towards a comprehensive model of change. In: Miller WR, Heather N (eds) *Treating Addictive Behaviours: Process of change*. Plenum, New York

SILAGY C, MANT D, FOWLER G et al. (1994) Meta-analysis on efficacy of nicotine replacement therapies in smoking cessation. *Lancet* **343**: 139–42

TASHKIN D, KANNER R, BAILEY W et al. (2001) Smoking cessation in patients with chronic obstructive pulmonary disease: a double-blind, placebo-controlled randomised trial. *Lancet* **357**: 1571–5

WEST R, McNEILL A, RAW M (2000) Smoking cessation guidelines for health professionals: an update. *Thorax* **55**: 987–99

7 Pharmacotherapy

BRONCHODILATORS

Main points

1 Bronchodilators are the most important treatment for symptom relief in COPD.

2 They work by
 – decreasing bronchomotor tone,
 – decreasing lung hyperinflation,
 – decreasing the work of breathing.

3 They are most appropriately taken by inhalation, and have a rapid onset of action.

4 An inhaler device should be selected that the patient can use effectively.

5 The patient's inhaler technique should be checked at regular intervals.

6 Short-acting beta-2 agonists and anticholinergics are equally efficacious. Sometimes combined therapy may have an additive effect.

7 In severe COPD, bronchodilators should be taken regularly four-hourly. In some patients, higher doses may prove more beneficial.

8 If symptomatic control is inadequate, adding one of the following should be considered:
 – long-acting beta-2 agonists,
 – long-acting anticholinergics,
 – theophyllines.

> Long-acting beta-2 agonists may improve quality of life
> and reduce the frequency of acute exacerbations.
> The new long-acting anticholinergic, tiotropium, has
> similar benefits and is taken once daily.
>
> **9** A small number of patients with severe COPD warrant a
> nebuliser trial.

Bronchodilators are the most important treatment in COPD. They form the cornerstone of therapy to improve symptoms and treat any reversible component of airflow obstruction.

The new NICE guidelines, in common with other international guidelines (except the current version of GOLD, which will shortly adopt the same standards), state that routine reversibility testing to bronchodilators and corticosteroids is no longer necessary (see also Chapter 11). Formal reversibility testing can be inconsistent within the same individual on different occasions and the often small changes seen may hide worthwhile symptomatic improvements gained by less easily measured areas of lung function. However, NICE does suggest that reversibility can be of value, particularly where there is doubt about differentiating COPD from asthma. A reversibility test to a single dose of bronchodilator that achieves a large improvement in lung function (more than 400ml in FEV_1) will help to identify patients with a significant asthmatic component to their disease.

Although reversibility testing can be part of the diagnostic process, a small or minimal change in lung function after a bronchodilator is not always a good predictor of the symptomatic improvement that patients might experience. It is therefore most important to prescribe a trial of bronchodilators, either beta-2 agonist or anticholinergic inhalers, to be used regularly for three to four weeks. Such trials must be performed when the patient is stable.

The symptomatic response described by the patient will help to determine both the efficacy of treatment and which bronchodilator provides most improvement. Patients frequently notice:

- a decrease in shortness of breath,

- improved walking distance,

- an overall better quality of life.

The most clinically useful way of assessing the response to a trial of inhaled therapy is to ask patients the five questions formulated by Paul Jones and others, listed in Chapter 5.

How do bronchodilators work?

Bronchodilators reverse the increased bronchomotor tone found in the airways of COPD patients by relaxing smooth muscle and thus reducing airway resistance. Several studies have shown improvements in vital capacity (VC) of 500ml or more, with a similar decrease in residual volume (RV) (see Chapter 4 and Figure 4.11). Hyperinflation is reduced, and it is easier and more comfortable for the patient to breathe. Breathlessness and the effort of breathing are reduced, so patients can walk further.

Beta-2 agonists also promote an increase in mucociliary activity, although the clinical importance of this is unclear. Theophyllines may, in addition, have a small effect on increasing respiratory muscle endurance, but again it is hard to assess whether this is of clinical significance.

Beta-2 agonists in high doses may also dilate pulmonary blood vessels. When ventilation of the lungs is impaired, as in acute exacerbations, this effect may cause a worsening of any ventilation/perfusion mismatch and result in a small, transient fall in arterial oxygen levels.

Bronchodilator administration

As in asthma, the preferred way to use a bronchodilator is by inhalation. Although oral bronchodilators may be just as effective in providing symptom relief, they have the disadvantages of greater side-effects, potential drug interactions and a slower onset of action.

Metered dose inhalers (MDIs) are inexpensive and effective, working rapidly to provide symptom relief. Correct timing and co-ordination can make them difficult to use, and less than 50% of patients can inhale from them effectively. This is especially so in elderly patients, who may have other illnesses such as arthritis or dementia. With repeated tuition, or the addition of a large volume spacer or breath-activated MDI, the proportion of patients able to use MDIs effectively can be greatly increased.

Dry powder devices are simpler to use and equally effective but are more expensive. As in asthma, it is essential that patients are prescribed a device that they can use effectively and are assessed regularly for competence in its use. Patients should be involved in the initial choice of device.

Short-acting bronchodilators

Short-acting beta-2 agonists: salbutamol and terbutaline

These drugs have a rapid onset of action (usually within five minutes) and a duration of action of three to four hours, and are recommended for both regular treatment and 'as required' for relief of symptoms. They can also be used before exercise to increase exercise tolerance or to relieve breathlessness. More severe levels of airflow obstruction should be treated with beta-2 agonists four-hourly (or even more frequently in extreme cases). It is safe and sometimes more effective to give two or three times the standard dose to achieve a better therapeutic response.

The regular use of short-acting beta-2 agonists in severe COPD is thus quite different from the accepted policy for all but the most severe grades of asthma (steps 4 and 5 in the BTS and SIGN British guidelines for asthma management), for which it is taught that they should be used only as required for symptom relief. As with any therapy, success or failure of a given agent should be assessed subjectively, from the point of view of the patient's perceived response over a month of treatment, and perhaps also objectively with lung function if appropriate. Alternatives or additions may then need to be explored.

Short-acting anticholinergic agent: ipratropium

Some older patients may become less responsive to beta-2 agonists and may achieve a better improvement with an anticholinergic agent. Short-acting anticholinergics have a slower onset of action (15–30 minutes) than short-acting beta-2 agonists (5 minutes) but the results of most comparative studies suggest that they are equally effective in achieving symptom relief. Indeed, in some they have produced a greater response and a longer duration of bronchodilation. The responses of individual patients to both anticholinergic and short-acting beta-2 agonist bronchodilators should therefore be assessed.

Combined short-acting therapy: salbutamol and ipratropium

The use of a short-acting beta-2 agonist with an anticholinergic may have an additive effect in some patients. Combined therapy may produce greater improvements in exercise tolerance and a greater degree of bronchodilation than either drug used separately.

If patients' symptoms improve with a combination of salbutamol and ipratropium, there is a clinical advantage in giving the drugs in a combined inhaler. Patients may find this more convenient and compliance may be enhanced.

Long-acting inhaled bronchodilators

Long-acting beta-2 agonists: salmeterol and formoterol

Long-acting beta-2 agonists have a duration of action of 12 hours, so they should be taken twice daily and on a regular basis to achieve the optimal effect. In asthma they provide good symptom relief, reduce acute exacerbations and much improve overall quality of life when added to mid to higher doses of inhaled steroids. Over the last few years there has been a considerable body of studies, including a Cochrane review, which have helped to clarify the role of long-acting beta-2 agonists in COPD. There have been more studies for salmeterol than formoterol but it seems that the two agents share many clinical actions.

Their effects on lung function are similar to those of short-acting beta-2 agonists in that there are some increases in FEV_1 and peak flow, larger increases in FVC and falls in residual volume, suggesting reduced hyperinflation. These actions continue for 12 hours compared with about 4 hours for the short-acting agents. Patients experience reductions in breathlessness, better exercise tolerance and, most important, a significant and sustained improvement in quality of life scores in both the total and symptom domains as judged by the St George's Respiratory Questionnaire. Salmeterol has also been shown to improve breathlessness at night and, in a study by Mahler and colleagues, to extend the time to the next acute exacerbation when compared with a placebo and ipratropium.

The short-term effects of long-acting beta-2 agonists are therefore similar to those of short-acting agents in improving lung function. In addition, there seems to be more sustained symptom improvement and significant benefit in health status that does not occur with the short-acting agents. In a recent review article, Johnson and Rennard have offered some possible explanations for the added properties of salmeterol. These observations are based on studies in vitro but may go part way to rationalising the extra properties of long-acting beta-2 agonists.

Salmeterol seems to protect airway epithelial cells from the damaging effect of bacteria such as *Haemophilus influenzae*. It improves cilial beat frequency and thus improves the clearance of mucus from the lungs. Salmeterol improves neutrophil function in several ways, which may help reduce the frequency of acute exacerbations.

More information is required to relate the clinical importance of these findings but long-acting beta-2 agonists have a useful role in COPD management, particularly if further studies confirm their ability to extend the time between exacerbations. Like other agents, they should have a clinical trial for four to eight weeks and be continued only if they are beneficial for the individual.

Long-acting anticholinergic: tiotropium

Tiotropium is a new selective antimuscarinic blocking agent that is inhaled as a dry powder once a day. It has some shared actions with ipratropium but binds mainly to the M3 airway receptors, which greatly enhances its activity and duration of action to 24 hours compared with 4–6 hours for ipratropium.

Tiotropium produced worthwhile increases in FEV_1 (over 100ml), FVC and PEF with no loss of efficacy over the three-month trial period, and the mean increase in FEV_1 was significantly greater than with ipratropium taken over a 24-hour period. Tiotropium also helped to reduce the number of exacerbations compared with ipratropium and helped reduce the decline in health status associated with increasing exacerbations.

A one-year study against placebo (Casaburi et al. 2002) confirmed worthwhile improvements in FEV_1, FVC and peak flow throughout the study period. Breathlessness was reduced and health status improved, 49% of patients on active therapy achieving at least a 4-point clinically meaningful increase on the overall score with the St George's Respiratory Questionnaire. There was a 14% reduction in exacerbations compared with placebo and a 47% reduction in hospitalisations. The time to first exacerbation was also significantly longer. A similar study for one year against ipratropium obtained similar results.

Oral long-acting bronchodilators

Beta-2 agonists

Generally these agents are not encouraged, as the inhaled versions work more rapidly and are safer. However, they may occasionally be justified for a patient with severe COPD who has difficulty using any form of inhaled therapy. If they are used, care must be taken to ensure that there is no significant side-effect such as tremor, tachycardia or hypokalaemia and that coexisting angina is not being made worse.

Theophyllines

Theophyllines produce only small amounts of bronchodilation in COPD and tend to be most effective in the higher parts of the narrow therapeutic range (i.e. blood levels of 10–20mg/litre). They can increase exercise tolerance, and some patients report a good improvement in symptoms. Other effects reported in research studies – such as an anti-inflammatory action, improvements in respiratory muscle strength and improvements in right ventricular performance – are difficult to evaluate clinically. If theophyllines are used, it is preferable to give them in a slow-release form, and to monitor serum theophylline levels regularly.

Side-effects such as nausea, headache and palpitations are common and there are also interactions with anti-epileptic drugs, diltiazem, verapamil, frusemide, erythromycin, ciprofloxacin and cimetidine, to name but a few. Blood levels are also influenced by smoking, viral infections, influenza vaccination and impaired renal and hepatic function. In elderly patients with multiple co-pathologies it can be extremely difficult to achieve an effective and stable blood level of theophylline. The risk/benefit ratio must therefore be considered carefully.

Nebulised bronchodilators

A small number of patients with severe COPD do not show any symptomatic improvement with inhaled bronchodilators, even with multiple doses taken through a large volume spacer. Sometimes benefit can be achieved only by using higher doses via a nebuliser. Nebulised bronchodilators are generally more expensive. They are also less convenient to administer because they take longer and a power source is usually required, although some nebuliser/compressor systems have rechargeable battery packs or run off a car cigarette lighter thus allowing the patient greater flexibility and mobility.

Nebuliser therapy

Nebulisers are devices that convert a drug solution into a continuous fine aerosol of sufficiently small particle size to penetrate to all levels of the airways. Drug inhalation is achieved by the patient breathing normally (tidal breathing) through the nebuliser over a five to ten minute period. The advantage of a nebuliser is that it can deliver a large dose of drug simply, particularly to patients who are too breathless or unwell to use a normal inhaler device effectively, or who have benefited clinically from higher doses.

The most commonly used varieties of nebuliser are:

- the standard jet nebuliser,
- the more advanced and efficient breath-assisted nebulisers, such as the Ventstream,
- the ultrasonic nebuliser,
- the mesh nebuliser.

The first two of these need to be driven by a compressor delivering flow rates of 6–8 litres per minute. A recent innovation, adaptive aerosol delivery, delivers the drug during inhalation only, thus eliminating waste of drug during exhalation, and can be programmed to deliver a precise dose. It costs more than both the standard nebuliser/compressor system and the ultrasonic nebuliser. If delivery of a precise amount of drug is not of paramount importance, it may not be a cost-effective option.

Ultrasonic and mesh nebuliser systems are smaller and operate almost silently. They are only suitable for single-patient use and are a little more expensive than the jet nebuliser systems. However, for a patient who requires a small, discreet system that is easy to use outside the home, these may be an attractive option.

The ultrasonic nebuliser uses ultrasound to agitate the drug solution so that droplets of appropriate size break off the surface. In the mesh system, drug solution is forced through microscopic holes in a metal mesh, forming respirable droplets of the solution. The mesh system is completely silent and very quick and efficient.

A mouthpiece is usually preferred to a facemask to deliver the nebulised mist. This is because there is a small risk of precipitating glaucoma when ipratropium or a combination of ipratropium and salbutamol is used via a facemask.

If a nebuliser/compressor system is supplied for long-term use at home, patients and their carers need to be given written instructions about cleaning and maintaining the equipment. Nebuliser chamber and mouthpiece or facemask need to be washed in warm soapy water and dried thoroughly after each use. The small jet holes in a jet nebuliser can be dried by attaching the nebuliser to the compressor and running the compressor for about ten seconds to remove any residual fluid. Standard disposable nebuliser chambers will last a single patient for three months of regular use before they become inefficient and need to be replaced. Tubing should not be washed inside because it is impossible to dry it effectively. Nebuliser equipment that is stored damp may constitute an infection risk.

Compressors need to be serviced regularly, according to manufacturer's instructions. An annual electrical safety check is the legal responsibility of whoever supplies the compressor. When compressor systems are supplied by a pharmaceutical company on a named patient basis, it is the responsibility of the doctor who recommended it to ensure that it is electrically safe.

In the surgery, standard nebulisers, tubing and masks are for single use only and should then be discarded. It is not possible to sterilise them effectively and there is thus a risk of passing infection from one patient to another. For medico-legal purposes, it is advisable to adhere to the single-use policy. 'Durable' nebulisers are made by some manufacturers; these can be sterilised effectively in an autoclave and used for a year. They may be more cost-effective than single-use disposable nebulisers. Maintenance of equipment should follow the manufacturer's recommendations.

Nebuliser trials

The BTS *Nebuliser Guidelines* require patients to attempt high-dose bronchodilator therapy with up to six to eight puffs four-hourly through a large volume spacer before undertaking a formal nebuliser trial. Multiple 'puffs' of bronchodilator are given through a spacer, with the patient inhaling each puff separately. Assessment for the appropriate use of a nebuliser should follow BTS Guidelines for nebuliser therapy and be carried out by a hospital specialist or a GP with experience of nebuliser trials. Nebulised beta-2 agonists and anticholinergics should be tried alone and then in combination in order to determine which therapy produces the best effect.

To perform a nebuliser trial the patient should be clinically stable. A suggested protocol is:

- Weeks 1–2: large volume spacer and high-dose bronchodilator

- Weeks 3–4: nebulised short-acting beta-2 agonist (e.g. salbutamol 2.5–5mg or terbutaline 5–10mg four times a day)

- Weeks 5–6: nebulised anticholinergic (e.g. ipratropium bromide 250–500μg four times a day)

- Weeks 7–8: nebulised combined short-acting beta-2 agonist and anticholinergic (e.g. salbutamol 5mg + ipratropium 500μg four times a day)

Patients should perform serial peak flow tests during the trial. A positive response is either an increase in lung function (improvement of 15% in peak flow during the trial) or a definite improvement in symptoms on active treatment. If a nebuliser is helpful, a nebuliser/compressor unit should be provided by the local chest clinic, who will:

- educate the patient and their carer(s) in its use,

- provide regular maintenance of the unit,

- supply disposables such as the nebuliser chamber, and

- provide emergency back-up in the event of breakdown.

Unfortunately, the provision of properly organised, hospital-based nebuliser services is patchy at best. In many areas of the UK, patients (or their GPs) are expected to purchase and maintain nebulisers for long-term use. This situation is far from satisfactory.

Bronchodilator therapy can improve a COPD patient's symptoms without necessarily producing significant changes in lung function. All patients should undergo therapeutic trials with different bronchodilators and different combinations of bronchodilators at different doses in order to determine which drug (or drugs) produces the best therapeutic response.

Further reading

General

BRITISH THORACIC SOCIETY (1997) BTS Guidelines for the management of chronic obstructive pulmonary disease. *Thorax* **52** (Suppl 5): S1–28

BRITISH THORACIC SOCIETY (1997) Current best practice for nebuliser treatment. *Thorax* **52** (Suppl 2): S1–106

NISAR M, WALSHAW M, EARIS JE, PEARSON M, CALVERLEY PMA (1990) Assessment of reversibility of airway obstruction in patients with chronic obstructive airways disease. *Thorax* **45**: 190–4.

Short-acting beta-2 agonists

BELLAMY D, HUTCHISON DCS (1981) The effects of salbutamol aerosol on the lung function of patients with emphysema. *British Journal of Diseases of the Chest* **75**: 190–5

VAN SCHAYCK CP, DOMPELING E, VAN HERWAARDEN CLA, FOLGERING H, VERBEEK AL, VAN DER HOOGEN HJ (1991) Bronchodilator treatment in moderate asthma or chronic bronchitis; continuous or on demand. A randomised controlled study. *British Medical Journal* **303**: 1426–31

Anticholinergics

ANTHONISEN NR, CONNETT JE, KILEY JP et al. (1994) Effects of smoking intervention and the use of an inhaled anticholinergic bronchodilator on the rate of decline of FEV₁. *Journal of the American Medical Association* **272**: 1497–505

BRAUN SR, McKENZIE WN, COPELAND C, KNIGHT I, ELLERSIECK M (1989) A comparison of the effect of ipratropium and albuterol in the treatment of chronic airways disease. *Archives of Internal Medicine* **149**: 544–7

COMBIVENT INHALATION AEROSOL STUDY (1994) Combination of ipratropium and albuterol is more effective than either agent alone. *Chest* **105**: 1411–19

LITTNER MR, ILOWITE JS, TASHKIN DA et al. (2000) Long-acting bronchodilation with once daily dosing of tiotropium in stable COPD. *American Journal of Respiratory and Critical Care Medicine* **161**: 1136–42

VAN NOORD JA, BANTJE TA, ELAND ME et al. (2000) A randomised controlled comparison of tiotropium and ipratropium in the treatment of COPD. *Thorax* **55**: 289–94

Long-acting beta-2 agonists

BOYD G, MORICE AH, POUNDSFORD JC, SIEBERT M, PESLIS N, CRAWFORD C (1997) An evaluation of salmeterol in the treatment of chronic obstructive airways disease. *European Respiratory Journal* **10**: 815–21

JOHNSON M, RENNARD S (2001) Alternative mechanisms for long-acting beta-2-adrenergic agonists in COPD. *Chest* **120**: 258–70

JONES PW, BOSH TK (1997) Quality of life changes in COPD patients treated with salmeterol. *American Journal of Respiratory and Critical Care Medicine* **155**: 1283–9

MAHLER DA, DONOHUE JF, BARBEE RA et al. (1999) Efficacy of salmeterol in the treatment of COPD. *Chest* **115**: 957–65

Long-acting anticholinergics

CASABURI R, MAHLER DA, JONES PW et al. (2002) A long-term evaluation of once-daily inhaled tiotropium in chronic obstructive pulmonary disease. *European Respiratory Journal* **19**: 217–24

VINCKEN W, VAN NOORD APM, GREEFHORST TA et al. (2002)
Improved health outcomes in patients with COPD during
1 year's treatment with tiotropium. *European Respiratory
Journal* **19**: 209–16

Theophyllines

McKAY SE, HOWIE CA, THOMSON AH, WHITING B, ADDIS GJ
(1993) Value of theophylline treatment in patients handicapped
by chronic obstructive pulmonary disease. *Thorax* **48**: 227–32

CORTICOSTEROID THERAPY

Main points

1 Inflammatory changes exist in the airways of patients with
COPD, with increases in neutrophils, T-lymphocytes and
macrophages. These inflammatory changes are different
from those in asthma.

2 The effect of inhaled corticosteroids on the various cells in
the airways has been inadequately studied.

3 The NICE guidelines state that corticosteroid reversibility
testing is not required for all patients on a routine basis.
When there is diagnostic doubt, a trial of prednisolone
30mg per day for two weeks should be done – an increase
greater than 400ml in FEV_1 is suggestive of asthma.

4 The GOLD guidelines still suggest that it is preferable to
perform steroid reversibility testing by giving an inhaled
challenge with beclometasone 1000µg per day (or
equivalent) for six weeks to three months, with objective
lung function measurement to assess responsiveness. This
may change in future GOLD guidelines.

5 Inhaled corticosteroids may produce an initial improvement in the first three to six months but have no effect on subsequent rate of decline in FEV_1.

6 The NICE and GOLD guidelines and the Royal College of Physicians of Edinburgh Consensus on COPD management suggest that patients with moderate to severe COPD, based on FEV_1% predicted, together with the presence of frequent exacerbations, constitute a positive indication for using regular (high dose) inhaled steroids. These patients do not require a steroid challenge to determine the efficacy of continuing inhaled therapy.

7 There is a lack of evidence to support the use of inhaled steroids in patients with mild disease.

8 When assessing the efficacy of corticosteroids, changes in symptoms, exacerbation frequency and health status should be considered just as much as FEV_1.

9 The Isolde study indicates that high-dose inhaled steroids improve clinical symptoms over three years, but the effect on the decline in lung function is less impressive. The Euroscop and Copenhagen long-term studies failed to show a clinically meaningful response or a significant improvement in lung function.

10 A meta-analysis of the effect of inhaled corticosteroids on lung function over two years suggests a small improvement in the treated group compared with those given a placebo, but only at high dosage. This might help to explain the differences in response between the large studies (Euroscop and Isolde), and perhaps indicates that high doses will be required to effect a worthwhile result. This dose-related effect was noted in early studies using oral steroids.

11 These important inhaled corticosteroid studies are first summarised below, and then followed by a more detailed appraisal.

In asthma, there is abundant evidence that the chronic inflammatory changes in the mucosa of the airways can be made histologically normal with both oral and inhaled corticosteroids. However, although the symptoms of most patients with COPD will improve with bronchodilator therapy, their response to corticosteroids is far less clear-cut. Although chronic inflammation is present in the small airways, there is little histological evidence of the effects that steroids may have on it. The situation is complicated because COPD is a spectrum of diseases ranging from the more obvious inflammation of chronic bronchitis to the destructive changes in the alveoli and supportive tissues in emphysema. Responses to steroid treatment will vary accordingly.

The rationale for using corticosteroids

The chronic inflammatory changes in the small airways of patients with COPD include increases both in the number of neutrophils and lymphocytes and in the number and activity of alveolar macrophages. The neutrophil is thought to be the most important cell in the pathogenesis of lung damage. Smokers with normal lung function often have increased neutrophils and macrophages.

The inflammation in asthma is characterised by thickening of the basement membrane as well as increased eosinophils and mast cells. These changes are not found in COPD, which suggests a different type of inflammatory process.

The NICE guidelines advice on inhaled steroids in COPD

Oral corticosteroid reversibility tests do not predict response to inhaled corticosteroid therapy and should not be used to identify which patients should be prescribed inhaled corticosteroids (evidence A). When there is diagnostic doubt, a trial of prednisolone 30mg per day for two weeks should be done – an increase greater than 400ml in FEV_1 is suggestive of asthma.

Inhaled corticosteroids should be prescribed for patients with an FEV_1 less than or equal to 50% predicted who have had two or more exacerbations in the last year. The aim of treatment is to reduce exacerbations and slow the rate of decline in health status, and not to slow the rate of decline in lung function (evidence B).

Clinicians should be aware, and patients informed, of the potential risk of developing osteoporosis and other side effects in people treated with high-dose inhaled corticosteroids (especially in the presence of other risk factors for osteoporosis).

New clinical information on inhaled steroids

A number of important studies on the action and response to inhaled steroids in COPD have been published since 1998. When evaluating the results of trials and studies, therefore, it is important to look at the outcomes being measured. For example:

- An improvement in symptoms and in quality of life.

- A reduction in the number of exacerbations.

- An improvement in lung function in the short term (six months).

- Slowing the rate of decline of lung function in the longer term (usually over three years).

- No benefit from inhaled steroids in milder disease.

There may be a small reduction in the risk of mortality for patients on long-term inhaled steroids (Sin and Tu 2001) but more prospective controlled studies are needed to assess this.

Summary of the messages from the new studies

- In the short term, there are clinically significant improvements in lung function and symptoms, with fewer acute exacerbations. The results from the Isolde study indicate that these improvements are maintained for three years.

- There is relatively little or no change in the rate of decline of lung function (FEV_1) over three years with various inhaled steroids in moderate to high dosage (Euroscop, Isolde, Copenhagen Lung Study, Lung Health 2 and the 1999 meta-analysis).

- Two recent meta-analyses (Highland et al. 2003, Sutherland et al. 2003), essentially analysing the same data from six studies, concluded that inhaled steroids, particularly in higher dose over two years had a small beneficial effect by reducing the rate of decline in FEV_1 by 9.9ml per year compared with placebo. The study by Highland et al. found the benefit to be only 5ml per year, which was not statistically significant. Where does this guide us? The inference is that inhaled steroids in high dosage may have a small benefit on reducing the rate of decline in lung function but seemingly not in patients with milder cases. The dose of inhaled steroid to be used in everyday practice remains uncertain but is probably in the region of beclometasone 800–1000µg per day, or equivalent.

■ The decline in quality of life is significantly slowed over a three-year period by high-dose fluticasone (Isolde).

■ The more positive clinical responses tend to occur only with higher dose inhaled steroids (meta-analysis, Isolde).

What are the implications for primary care?

The results of the studies suggest that inhaled steroids have minimal effect on the long-term decline of lung function, and that the very small changes reported from some studies may or may not be clinically beneficial. However, there is growing evidence indicating worthwhile improvement in health status and symptoms and a reduction in the number of exacerbations. This is of considerable interest to patients.

As often happens with major studies that set out to answer important clinical questions, the results sometimes raise further issues and questions about how to treat patients. Some of the questions include:

■ Isolde used high-dose fluticasone (1000µg per day). Would a smaller dose have the same effect?

■ At what stage should patients be given inhaled steroids – more, certainly, with severe symptoms and exacerbations but what about for less severe symptoms?

■ Do the benefits of reduced exacerbations and symptoms balance the cost and possible side-effects of high-dose inhaled steroids?

■ Is there some way of identifying sub-groups of patients who are more likely to benefit from treatment? COPD is a heterogeneous spectrum of pathologies and perhaps patients with greater degrees of reversibility might do better?

Is there a role for long-term oral steroids?

Most GP practices have patients with severe COPD who take oral steroids, usually for acute exacerbations. However, because of the potential side-effects, the NICE guidelines do not recommend the regular use of oral steroids. When the steroids are gradually stopped, the patient may deteriorate rapidly, with worsening dyspnoea, cough or wheeze. So a further course of steroids is given. If the symptoms become worse as the steroids are again reduced, this usually indicates the need for ongoing oral steroid therapy. Such circumstances usually guide the decision to continue oral steroids unless or until their side-effects outweigh the benefits. Each patient needs to be counselled about the advantages and disadvantages of steroid therapy in relation to the severity of their disease, likely benefits and the side-effects, and should be involved in the decision whether to continue.

The likelihood of serious side-effects is fairly small when a low dose of oral steroids is used. Each patient should be observed carefully for reduced mobility due to muscle weakness in the thighs from steroid myopathy.

A number of guidelines have appeared relating to the increased risk of bone fracture with oral steroids. Vertebral fractures are more likely to occur than limb fractures; they are related to the steroid dose but also to risk factors particular to the individual patient. As the greatest rate of bone loss seems to happen in the first 12 months of treatment, early steps to prevent osteoporosis are important.

One of the guidelines uses a dose of 5mg per day as a cut-off point and recommends that bone mineral density be measured by dexa-scan above this threshold. Recommended treatment is with bisphosphonates, which significantly increase bone density but, according to a Cochrane review, do not reduce overall fractures.

Steroids for acute exacerbations

It is common practice in primary and secondary care to treat exacerbations of COPD with courses of prednisolone, particularly when the symptoms are increasing breathlessness, wheeze and chest tightness. Symptoms usually return to baseline levels over one to three weeks and, as with acute asthma, the steroid treatment may need to be continued for up to 14 days.

Do corticosteroids have particular side-effects in COPD?

The side-effects of inhaled and systemic steroids are summarised in Table 7.1. Four factors are relevant to the use of corticosteroids in COPD:

- Patients are generally older.

- Most patients have a significant smoking history.

- Those with severe COPD have a limited life expectancy.

- Most receive a relatively small dose of corticosteroid.

Inhaled steroids seem to cause only minor side-effects, apart from mild oral and laryngeal problems and an increased risk of bruising. Oral steroids cause suppression of pituitary–adrenal function but this side-effect is probably of little clinical importance. Perhaps the main concern in severe COPD is the potential added effect on bone thinning from smoking and inactivity. Unfortunately, there have not been any controlled studies that specifically addressed these questions.

Table 7.1 Side-effects of corticosteroids

Inhaled	*Systemic*
Oral candidiasis	Suppressed hypothalamic–pituitary–adrenal function
Dysphonia	Osteoporosis
Bruising	Hypertension
?Cataracts	Cataracts
	Weight gain
	Dyspepsia
	Cushingoid appearance
	Mood change
	Peripheral oedema
	Risk of diabetes
	Myopathy

Synopsis of important clinical trials of inhaled steroids in COPD

Short-term trials

The study of **Dompeling et al.** (1992) examined a mixed group of asthma and COPD patients with known more rapid decline in lung function than usual. All patients were treated for a year with beclometasone 800µg daily together with either salbutamol or ipratropium. In the patients with COPD there was a significant improvement in the rate of decline of FEV_1 in the first six months of treatment, but from months 7 to 12 the rate of decline returned to pre-steroid treatment levels. There was no change in the number of exacerbations but a small improvement in the symptoms of cough, sputum and dyspnoea. This study thus suggests small improvements in symptoms and slowed rate of decline in FEV_1 in the first six months that subsequently revert to pre-steroid treatment levels.

The two-year study by **Renkema et al.** (1996) examined 58 non-allergic patients with COPD. They were given:

- budesonide 1600µg per day, or

- budesonide 1600µg per day plus oral prednisolone 5mg per day, or

- a placebo.

As with the Dompeling study, there was a small but significant improvement in symptoms but no change in the number of exacerbations. The rate of decline of FEV_1 was:

- budesonide only: 30ml per year,

- budesonide plus prednisolone: 40ml per year,

- placebo: 60ml per year.

Because of a wide scatter of results, none of the differences reached statistical significance. The authors concluded that, over all, the benefits of the steroids were small but that some patients might achieve worthwhile responses. More studies are required to determine which COPD patients should receive inhaled steroids.

A multi-centre study by **Paggiaro et al.** (1998) compared fluticasone 1000µg per day with a placebo in 281 patients over a six-month period. These patients generally had more severe COPD than those in the studies described above. Outcome measures were symptom scores, exacerbations and lung function. Compared with the placebo group, the active treatment group had:

- fewer exacerbations ($p < 0.001$),

- improved symptom scores,

- a greater walking distance,

- improved peak flow and FEV_1.

This study also indicates a short-term improvement with inhaled corticosteroids, but the dose of fluticasone was high and probably more than would customarily be used in general practice. We do not know whether this response would have continued if the study had been extended although a longer study, Isolde, gives some indication (see later).

In complete contrast, a study from Canada by **Bourbeau et al.** (1998) has shown no response to budesonide 1600µg per day over six months. This was also a placebo-controlled trial but the patients included had severe, advanced COPD. Initially, all patients received prednisolone 40mg per day for two weeks, and only those who were deemed steroid non-responders entered the double-blind phase of the study. Only 13.5% of the original 140 patients were designated steroid responders. There were no differences in FEV_1, symptom scores or quality of life scores between the treatment and the placebo groups.

These studies help to demonstrate the difficulty in interpreting the efficacy of inhaled steroids and the importance of knowing the selection criteria for the patients studied. The Dompeling study had patients with milder COPD; moreover, some of them were atopic and thus more likely to respond to the steroid. Over all, though, there seems to be a favourable short-term effect on symptoms in the first six months. The longer term changes in the rate of decline of lung function are, however, minimal.

Longer term studies

Two early studies by **Postma** (1985, 1988) reviewed retrospectively a group of patients with severe COPD for between 2 and 20 years. The patients who had regularly been taking oral prednisolone 10mg or more per day had a slower decline in FEV_1. If, however, the dose of prednisolone was reduced to less than 10mg per day, the FEV_1 tended to fall more rapidly. It is therefore important to balance the clinical benefits with the likely increasing number of side-effects from oral steroid therapy. At present, only patients with severe COPD would be considered for long-term oral steroids.

Multi-centre studies

Three major multi-centre studies have recently been completed. Each addressed the longer term effect of inhaled steroids on the decline of lung function compared with a control group.

Euroscop (Pauwels et al., 1999) was a large European placebo-controlled study examining the effect of budesonide 800μg per day on the rate of decline of lung function over a three-year period. Entry criteria to the study included being a current smoker with a FEV_1/FVC ratio less than 70% and less than 10% reversibility following a course of prednisolone. Initially, 2147 people were recruited; those who stopped smoking or were non-compliant during the run-in period were dropped from the study, leaving 1277 participants. They had a mean age of 52 years and a mean FEV_1% predicted of 77% – mild COPD. The primary outcome variable was post-bronchodilator FEV_1.

The results revealed relatively small differences between the two groups. The overall three-year decline in FEV_1 was 140ml in the budesonide group and 180ml in the placebo group.

As in other studies, there was an initial improvement over the first six months with the inhaled steroid, followed by a similar decline from 9 to 36 months. Subgroup analysis revealed that:

- women did better than men,

- heavier smokers declined more rapidly,

- atopy had no significant role.

The overall conclusion was that the inhaled steroid had a limited long-term benefit on the rate of decline in lung function.

Isolde (Burge et al., 2000) This British study compared fluticasone 500μg twice daily (via MDI and large volume spacer) with a placebo in moderate to severe COPD over a three-year period. The participants were older (mean age 64) and heavy smokers (44 pack-years). Outcome measures were:

- post-bronchodilator FEV_1,

- frequency of exacerbations,

- withdrawal from the study for respiratory reasons,

- health status scores.

After a two-month run-in period to obtain baseline levels, participants were given an oral prednisolone challenge and then randomised to fluticasone (376 patients, of whom 216 completed) or placebo (375 patients, of whom 180 completed). The mean FEV_1% predicted was 50% with steroid reversibility of 6%.

The difference in the *total rate of decline of FEV_1* over the three years was greater than in the Euroscop study, with values of 133ml for the fluticasone group and 197ml for the placebo group (p = 0.0003). In the fluticasone group, the improvement peaked at six to nine months. Thereafter the annual decline in FEV_1 was fairly similar at 50ml for fluticasone and 59ml for placebo.

Exacerbation rates were lower on fluticasone (0.99 per year vs 1.32 on placebo) and there were more *withdrawals for respiratory causes* in the placebo group.

Health status was assessed using the St George's Questionnaire, which correlates well with respiratory symptoms but less well with FEV_1. A significant clinical change on this scale corresponds to four 'units'. Participants receiving fluticasone had a significantly slower rate of decline in health status than did those on placebo. A deterioration of four units occurred every 15 months in the placebo group, against 24 months in the fluticasone group. Thus, in this study of patients with moderate to severe COPD, high-dose fluticasone resulted in fewer exacerbations, improved symptoms and a better quality of life throughout the period of the study. The effect on the rate of decline in lung function was small, particularly over the last two years of the study. The run-in phase of this study showed that a conventional oral corticosteroid trial was a poor predictor of the response to long-term inhaled corticosteroid therapy.

Copenhagen Lung Study (Vestbo et al., 1999) This three-year Danish study compared budesonide 800μg per day (via turbohaler) with a placebo. The patients recruited for it had very mild impairment of lung function (FEV_1% predicted 86%); indeed, many of them would not match the BTS Guidelines definition of COPD. However, they were all heavy smokers. Out of 416 patients, 395 had no response to an initial trial with prednisolone.

At the end of the study, the decline in FEV_1 was almost identical: 46ml per year for the group receiving budesonide and 49ml per year for the placebo group – indicating no significant clinical benefit from budesonide over three years. However, the selection of steroid non-responders and an initial six months of high-dose budesonide would minimise any effect.

Lung Health 2 Study (2000) This large study from the USA enrolled 1116 patients with milder COPD (mean FEV_1 of 68% predicted) and treated them with the inhaled steroid triamcinolone or a placebo for three years. The dose used was lower than that used in other studies. As with the other studies, there was no effect on the rate of decline of FEV_1 between the treatment groups. However, patients in the triamcinolone group had fewer respiratory symptoms and fewer visits to a respiratory physician. The side-effects were carefully monitored and revealed that the bone density in the steroid group decreased during the study. Triamcinolone is, however, recognised as a less selective inhaled steroid and is not used in this format in the UK.

Inhaled corticosteroid meta-analysis (Van Grunsven et al., 1999) This combined Dutch–French meta-analysis looked at the effects of inhaled steroids in placebo-controlled trials over a two-year period. It identified three studies – two published and one in abstract form – and reanalysed the original data to conform to a more uniform format. Patients were included only if they had definite COPD.

The results show a small improvement of FEV_1 of 34ml per year in favour of the group receiving inhaled steroids. There was no difference in exacerbation rates in the two groups. The patients in the studies using high-dose steroids (beclometasone 1500µg per day) did better than those on lower doses (budesonide 800µg per day), in whom there was little effect.

The authors of the paper conclude that this is the first published study to show a preservation of FEV_1 during two years of treatment, but only with high doses of inhaled steroid. This important study adds weight to the provisional early reports from the Isolde study that high-dose inhaled steroids seem to have a beneficial effect on long-term COPD; lower doses apparently do not.

Further reading

General

BRITISH THORACIC SOCIETY (1997) BTS Guidelines for the management of chronic obstructive pulmonary disease. *Thorax* **52**
(Suppl 5): S1–28

Common issues in osteoporosis. *MeReC Bulletin* (2001) **12**: 5–8

JARAD NA, WEDZICHA JA, BURGE PS et al. (1999) An
observational study of inhaled corticosteroid withdrawal in
stable chronic obstructive pulmonary disease. *Respiratory
Medicine* **93**: 161–6

MCEVOY CE, NIEWOEHNER DE (1997) Adverse effects of corticosteroid therapy for COPD – a critical review. *Chest* **111**: 732–43

ROYAL COLLEGE OF PHYSICIANS OF EDINBURGH (2001) *Consensus
Statement on the Management of COPD*. RCPE, Edinburgh
[Available on-line (contact details in the 'Useful addresses'
section)]

SIN DD, TU JV (2001) Inhaled corticosteroids and the risk of
mortality and readmission in elderly patients with COPD.
American Journal of Respiratory and Critical Care Medicine
164: 580–4

THOMPSON WH, NIELSON CP, CARVALHO P et al. (1996) Controlled
trial of oral prednisolone in outpatients with acute COPD
exacerbation. *American Journal of Respiratory and Critical Care
Medicine* **154**: 407–12

Short-term trials

BOURBEAU J, ROULEAU MY, BOUCHER S (1998) Randomised
controlled trial of inhaled corticosteroids in patients with
COPD. *Thorax* **53**: 447–82

DOMPELING E, VAN SCHAYK CP, MOLEMA J et al. (1992) Inhaled
beclometasone improves the course of asthma and COPD.
European Respiratory Journal **5**: 945–52

PAGGIARO PL, DAHLE R, BAKRAN I et al. (1998) Multicentre
randomised placebo controlled trial of inhaled fluticasone in
patients with COPD. *Lancet* **351**: 773–9

RENKEMA TEJ, SCHOUTEN MS, KOETER GH, POSTMA DS (1996)
Effects of long term treatment with corticosteroids in COPD.
Chest **109**: 1156–62

Long-term trials

BURGE PS, CALVERLEY PMA, JONES PW et al. (2000) Randomised, double-blind, placebo-controlled study of fluticasone propionate in patients with moderate to severe chronic obstructive pulmonary disease: the Isolde trial. *British Medical Journal* **320**: 1297–303

LUNG HEALTH STUDY RESEARCH GROUP (2000) Effect of inhaled triamcinolone on the decline in pulmonary function in COPD. *New England Journal of Medicine* **343**: 1902–9

PAUWELS RA, LOFDAHL C, LAITINEN LA et al. (1999) Long-term treatment with inhaled budesonide in persons with mild chronic obstructive pulmonary disease who continue smoking. *New England Journal of Medicine* **340**: 1948–53

POSTMA DS, STEENHUIS EJ, VANDERWEELE LT et al. (1985) Severe chronic airflow obstruction: can corticosteroids slow down progression? *European Journal of Respiratory Disease* **67**: 56–64

POSTMA DS, PETERS I, STEENHUIS EJ et al. (1988) Moderately severe chronic airflow obstruction: can corticosteroids slow down progression? *European Respiratory Journal* **1**: 22–6

VESTBO J, SORENSEN T, LANGE P et al. (1999) Long-term effects of inhaled budesonide in mild and moderate chronic obstructive pulmonary disease: a randomised controlled trial. *Lancet* **353**: 1819–23

Meta-analysis

HIGHLAND KB, STRANGE C, HEFFNER JE (2003) Long-term effects of inhaled corticosteroids on FEV_1 in patients with COPD. A meta-analysis. *Archives of Internal Medicine* **138**: 969–73

SUTHERLAND ER, ALLMERS H, AYAS NT et al. (2003) Inhaled corticosteroids reduce the progression of airflow obstruction in COPD; a meta-analysis. *Thorax* **58**: 937–41

VAN GRUNSVEN PM, VAN SCHAYCK CP, DERENNE JP et al. (1999) Long term effects of inhaled corticosteroids in chronic obstructive pulmonary disease: a meta-analysis. *Thorax* **54**: 7–14

COMBINED INHALED LONG-ACTING BETA-AGONISTS AND CORTICOSTEROIDS

Main point

The combination of inhaled steroid and long-acting beta-2 agonists achieves a better outcome than either drug used on its own.

Two forms of combined long-acting beta-agonists plus cortico-steroids have had additive effects in asthma, with clinical outcomes better than both agents given in the same dose but by separate inhalers. There have been at least four large studies in COPD that have shown consistent benefits in a range of outcome measures – which confirms the advantage of using both agents together.

Salmeterol/fluticasone studies

Mahler et al. (2002) carried out a six-month four-arm study with placebo, salmeterol, fluticasone 500µg twice daily and a combination of active drugs. All active treatments produced improvements in lung function and breathlessness, and a reduction in reliever therapy, but the combined drug achieved significantly greater change than either drug alone.

The **TRISTAN** study – the Trial of Inhaled Steroids and Long-Acting Beta-2 Agonists (**Calverley et al.** 2003a) – used the same design but was for one year and looked at other clinical outcomes. Lung function and symptom improvements mirrored those found by Mahler. In addition, the combined agent, but not the single drugs on their own, achieved a clinically meaningful improvement in health status greater than 4 points (St George's Respiratory Questionnaire; SGRQ) and a reduction in exacerbations, particularly in patients with more severe disease and an FEV_1 below 50% predicted.

Formoterol/budesonide studies

A one-year study by **Szafranski et al.** (2003) with a similar four-arm design used budesonide in the lower dose of 800µg per day in the combined and single inhaler. There were similar significant improvements for all active treatments, with greater lung function, reduced symptoms and an almost clinically significant change of 3.9 points on the SGRQ health status score. Exacerbations were reduced by 24% using the combined drug compared with placebo.

A further study by **Calverley et al.** (2003a, b) had a slightly different design: patients were given two weeks of prednisolone initially and then followed up for one year. Lung function with the combined therapy maintained the prednisolone-induced improvement while all other therapies declined towards baseline. The combined treatment further enhanced the improvement in the SGRQ score from 4 to 7 points with only mild deterioration in other active treatments. A reduction in exacerbation rate similar to that in the previous study was noted.

The combined results from these studies are very consistent and show added efficacy from combined agents. NICE also recommends such combinations as long as clinical efficacy is demonstrated for each patient.

Further reading

CALVERLEY P, PAUWELS R, VESTBO J et al. (2003a) Combined salmeterol and fluticasone in the treatment of chronic obstructive pulmonary disease: a randomised controlled trial (TRISTAN). *Lancet* **361**: 449–56

CALVERLEY PM, BOONSAWAT W, CSEKE Z et al. (2003b) Maintenance therapy with budesonide and formoterol in COPD. *European Respiratory Journal* **22**: 912–19

MAHLER DA, WIRE P, HORSTMAN D et al. (2002) Effectiveness of fluticasone and salmeterol combination delivered by the Diskus device in the treatment of COPD. *American Journal of Respiratory and Critical Care Medicine* **166**: 1084–91

SZAFRANSKI W, CUKIER A, RAMIREZ G et al. (2003) Efficacy and safety of budesonide/formoterol in the management of COPD. *European Respiratory Journal* **21**: 74–81

MUCOLYTICS

NICE has recommended that agents such as carbocisteine may be considered for patients with a chronic productive cough (evidence B).

Such drugs also have antoxidant properties and a Cochrane review of similar agents showed that they reduced exacerbations by 29% compared with placebo.

Further reading

POOLE P, BLACK PN (2001) Oral mucolytic drugs for exacerbations of chronic pulmonary disease: a systematic review. *British Medical Journal* **322**: 1271–4

8 | Pulmonary rehabilitation

Main points

1 Pulmonary rehabilitation has been shown to:
   – reduce breathlessness,
   – improve functional ability,
   – improve health-related quality of life.
2 Pulmonary rehabilitation may also lead to a reduction in use of the health service, in hospital admissions and in in-patient stays.
3 Rehabilitation should be available to *all* patients who feel they are functionally disabled by their COPD.
4 The cornerstone of rehabilitation is individually prescribed exercise endurance training.
5 Exercise for specific muscle groups can improve functional ability and may be particularly useful for patients with very severe disease.
6 Education about the disease and its management, nutrition, relaxation and coping strategies, and the management of exacerbations should also be included.
7 The patient's carer should be actively encouraged to be involved in the rehabilitation programme.
8 Support and encouragement to continue with lifestyle changes at the end of the programme are helpful.
9 *All patients benefit from keeping active.*

Historically, the management of COPD has focused on strategies either to prevent deterioration (stopping smoking) or to improve lung function (using bronchodilators and corticosteroids). Treatment that aimed to improve quality of life or health status and functional ability received little attention.

Now, however, there is increasing recognition that interventions can be made to improve patients' health status and to improve their ability to live with their condition. The nature of COPD – *fixed or partially fixed airflow obstruction* – means that improvement in lung function (impairment) can be at best modest, whereas improvement in patients' functional performance and health status (disability and handicap) can be considerable. Pulmonary rehabilitation focuses on these areas.

Evidence for the effectiveness of rehabilitation in COPD

A dictionary definition of rehabilitation is:

> 'to restore to good condition; to make fit after disablement or illness'.

Rehabilitation aims to restore the individual to the best physical, mental and emotional state possible. The ethos of rehabilitation has been embraced enthusiastically in the fields of cardiology, orthopaedics and neurology. In the UK, however, it has been adopted only slowly in respiratory medicine even though published guidelines from the European Respiratory Society, the American Thoracic Society and the British Thoracic Society and the global GOLD guidelines state that rehabilitation is an important part of COPD management. It is pleasing that the NICE guidelines state that rehabilitation should be offered and available to any COPD patient who feels they are disabled by their condition.

Whether pulmonary rehabilitation has an effect on mortality from COPD is controversial. It seems that the most important factor in determining survival is the post-bronchodilator FEV_1. However, maximal exercise capacity is also a factor in determining the prognosis in a patient with COPD, and pulmonary rehabilitation that improves maximal exercise capacity may also have a beneficial effect on mortality. It must be borne in mind, though, that extending the life of a COPD patient is not the prime aim of rehabilitation. Rather, it is to improve the quality and reduce the dependence of their remaining years.

There is plenty of evidence that pulmonary rehabilitation is effective in reducing breathlessness and improving exercise tolerance. Controlled studies have revealed that the sensation of dyspnoea is reduced and exercise capacity is increased after exercise training, and health-related quality of life scores also improve following rehabilitation programmes.

Evidence that pulmonary rehabilitation reduces the need for health care has come largely from the USA. There, programmes are sometimes eligible for reimbursement by insurers because they have been found to substantially reduce both hospital admission rates and inpatient stays. There has been little motivation to reduce the cost of emergency admissions for COPD in the UK but, with recent NHS reforms, this situation is likely to change. A survey by the British Thoracic Society and the British Lung Foundation in 2003 highlighted the lack of availability, resources and funding for pulmonary rehabilitation in the UK. It is hoped that the NICE guidelines will provide the spur to improve this situation. Obviously, the financial saving to the health service depends on the cost of the rehabilitation programme, but they are generally 'low tech' and cheap compared with the cost of admitting a patient to hospital because of an exacerbation of COPD.

Recent health economic data from UK centres have also confirmed that pulmonary rehabilitation is cost effective. Even when all indirect costs such as transport and carers' time off work have been taken into consideration, it costs no more to rehabilitate COPD patients than to treat them without rehabilitation. Patients are more likely to be admitted and will use more health services, in both primary and secondary care, than if they had undergone a programme of rehabilitation.

Why rehabilitation programmes are needed

Breathlessness on exertion and the fear, anxiety and panic it engenders often lead a person with COPD to avoid activity. Attacks of breathlessness or coughing that occur outside the home may cause particular anxiety and embarrassment. Exercise avoidance results in deconditioning of skeletal muscles and, in turn, increasing disability; COPD patients often report that the limiting factor to their exercise tolerance is tiredness in the legs rather than breathlessness. Avoiding exercise, as well as the fear that breathlessness invokes, leads to a general loss of confidence, sowing the seeds of social isolation and increasing dependence. Increasing inactivity and isolation further compound the problem and the patient is in a vicious circle that results in increasing dependence, disability and worsening quality of life (Figure 8.1.)

For many COPD patients the 'normal' irritations and stresses of

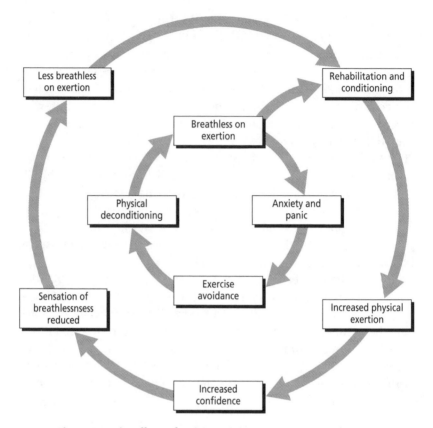

Figure 8.1 The effects of activity or inactivity on exercise tolerance.
(Reproduced by permission of the National Respiratory Training Centre)

everyday life are sufficient to induce breathlessness. The phenome-non of the 'emotional straitjacket' of advanced COPD is widely recognised.

- A passive dependent role may be adopted, in which the patient takes little part in family life.

- Patients feel they are a burden to their families.

- Frustration is often expressed as anger, usually directed at the family carer.

- Guilt at what is seen as a 'self-inflicted' disease is another common emotion.

■ Resentment on the part of the carer at the restrictions this disease imposes on long-held plans for retirement may also be manifest.

■ Self-destructive patterns of behaviour, such as a refusal to contemplate stopping smoking, are often seen.

■ Self-esteem is frequently very low, and depression is common.

■ Many patients refuse to exercise or will be restrained by an over-protective carer from exercising, even within their limited potential.

The aim of pulmonary rehabilitation is to break this vicious circle of increasing inactivity and breathlessness and to improve exercise capacity and functional ability.

The components of a hospital-based pulmonary rehabilitation programme

Pulmonary rehabilitation programmes usually consist of three main components:

■ exercise training,

■ education about the disease and its management,

■ psychosocial support.

Exercise

Exercise (aerobic) training to recondition skeletal muscles and improve exercise endurance forms the cornerstone of most programmes. The amount of exercise prescribed is determined on an individual basis and is based either on a laboratory treadmill or cycle ergometer test or a field exercise test, such as the relatively simple shuttle walking test (see Chapter 5). The shuttle walking test is closely related to an individual's peak oxygen consumption (Vo_2 peak) and allows a reasonably accurate prescription of exercise. It has been suggested that, when there is no access to exercise-testing equipment, patients may be able to determine their own training regimen, based on their perception of breathlessness. A Borg scale (see Table 5.4) is often employed, and the patient is encouraged to exercise to between levels 3 and 5 (moderate to severe).

Most hospital-based programmes use cycling or walking for exercise endurance training. Generally, an attempt is made to prescribe a form of regular exercise that the patient will find easy to continue at home both during and after the rehabilitation programme. Walking and cycling are also activities that have some meaning for the patient in terms of their daily lives.

Exercises that train specific groups of muscles, such as the upper limb girdle muscles, are usually included in a training programme and are aimed at improving the patient's ability to perform particular tasks associated with daily living. In someone with COPD the accessory muscles of respiration may be used. Any activity that uses the same muscle groups, such as brushing the hair or carrying shopping, is likely to increase the breathlessness. Specific exercises for particular muscle groups may be of great benefit for patients with severe COPD, who may find aerobic exercise too demanding. The exercises are generally of the more gentle bend-and-stretch variety, but may still give good results in increasing functional ability.

The role of respiratory muscle training in pulmonary rehabilitation is debatable. Training the respiratory muscles for strength and endurance has been successful in healthy subjects and in patients with chronic airflow obstruction but evidence that such training produces clinically significant results is equivocal. Further research is awaited.

Hospital pulmonary rehabilitation programmes are generally multidisciplinary and do not consist of exercise training alone. The first hour of a session is usually devoted to an exercise routine and the second hour to educating the patient and family about the disease, its management and how to develop strategies to live with it (summarised in Table 8.1). Partners and carers are generally actively encouraged to attend. A carer's need for information and social support is often as great as, if not greater than, the patient's.

Education and advice

People need basic information about the lungs in health and disease to help them understand the role of smoking in the development of COPD. Some centres exclude patients who continue to smoke but others will accept them and include smoking cessation in their education programme. There is certainly some logic to this approach. If smokers are excluded from rehabilitation, a low self-esteem – 'I'm

Table 8.1 Components of pulmonary rehabilitation

Exercise

Endurance (aerobic) training:
  Walking
  Cycling
Specific muscle groups (e.g. upper limb girdle)
?Respiratory muscle training (value debatable)

Education

The lungs in health and disease
Drug treatment
Self-management
Stopping smoking
Nutrition
Breathing control and sputum clearance
Relaxation techniques/coping strategies
Dealing with everyday activities
Financial support and benefits

not worth the trouble' – may well be reinforced. Joining a programme with other COPD sufferers who have successfully 'kicked the habit' may provide added incentive for an attempt to quit.

Advice is also given about the drug treatment of COPD and how to manage exacerbations effectively. Other professionals may be involved in giving additional education. For example:

- Dieticians can provide valuable general advice on healthy eating; they are also available to provide specific advice to the overweight or underweight patient.

- A physiotherapist can teach sputum clearance techniques and breathing control. Relaxation and coping skills are also valuable.

- The occupational therapist can provide advice or equipment to help with activities of daily living.

- The social worker may be able to give advice on benefits and financial matters.

Marital and sexual problems are common among these patients, so specialist help and advice may also be needed.

Psychosocial support

Many patients with advanced COPD are socially isolated. Pulmonary rehabilitation programmes can provide both patients and their partners/carers with valuable social contact. The support provided by group members can be enormous.

The setting of pulmonary rehabilitation and the personnel involved vary widely, depending very much on local circumstances. Some centres offer inpatient rehabilitation and in some areas home or primary-care-based programmes are available. A programme should consist of two or three sessions a week for six to eight weeks, combined with a programme of exercises the patient performs at home between sessions. The maintenance of improvement after a rehabilitation programme seems to be long-lasting but some sort of follow-up and after-care would probably be beneficial. Clearly, for this to be provided indefinitely in a hospital setting would be expensive and, it could be argued, might serve to undermine the philosophy of self-reliance that is engendered as part of the initial programme.

The provision of a 'training diary' or an occasional 'refresher' session is offered by some centres as a solution to the problem of continuing support. In others, patients 'graduate' from pulmonary rehabilitation to a patient support group. The British Lung Foundation's Breathe Easy groups provide an ideal forum for continuing social contact, support and encouragement. Some centres graduate less severely disabled patients to an 'exercise on prescription' group at local sports centres where they can still meet regularly, exercise and benefit from mutual support.

The role of the primary health care team

The provision of hospital-based rehabilitation programmes is far from uniform at present – despite increasing evidence of its efficacy and cost effectiveness. Where such schemes exist, the role of the primary health care team is:

- to select appropriate patients for referral,

- to support and encourage patients undergoing rehabilitation,

- to follow-up and provide continued encouragement for patients who have graduated from hospital programmes.

Table 8.2 Patient selection

Motivated to improve

On optimal treatment and compliant with treatment

Increasing disability

Clinically stable

Able to exercise (caution with cardiac, orthopaedic or neurological problems)

Before a referral for rehabilitation is considered, it should be ensured that the patient is on optimum therapy and that no further improvements with additional drug intervention can be achieved. It is also usual to refer patients in a period of clinical stability, although for those who have frequent exacerbations this may be difficult and referrals may be appropriate during a convalescent period. It is also important to consider whether the patient's disability is related solely to COPD or if there is a significant co-morbidity that will limit the effectiveness of rehabilitation. For example, a patient who has severe rheumatoid arthritis or ischaemic heart disease may be unable to undertake the exercise component of the programme. However, some centres will accept such patients for the education component of the programme.

The selection of appropriate patients is crucial and is not based solely on clinical criteria (Table 8.2):

- Current smokers might not be accepted, as discussed earlier. Some physicians consider that patients who are unable to stop smoking are unlikely to be able to make the lifestyle changes that are at the core of rehabilitation and are also unlikely to adhere to an exercise programme.

- Difficulties with travel may mean that ambulance transport will have to be arranged.

- If the patient is still working, there may be difficulties with attending all the sessions.

- Perhaps the most important consideration of all is *the patient's motivation to improve.*

If your area includes people from ethnic minorities, there may be language and culture difficulties. However, it may be possible to gather a group of patients of the same ethnic origin and use an interpreter who can also advise on cultural aspects.

The fact that a patient is using oxygen is not generally a reason to exclude them from a rehabilitation programme, and neither is the severity of their condition. It could be argued that patients with severe disease stand to gain the most from rehabilitation.

Where there are no formal rehabilitation programmes, the primary health care team may need to be innovative and enlist whatever services are available locally. Protected time in a structured COPD clinic in general practice can provide a useful forum for delivering basic education about COPD to patients and their carers. A community physiotherapist, particularly if they have a respiratory interest, may be a useful resource. Leaflets containing information about suitable gentle exercises and breathing control are available from the British Lung Foundation (see the 'Useful address' at the end of this chapter). Patients need to be reassured that getting breathless when exercising will not cause any further damage to their lungs, and they should all be encouraged to keep active and take some form of regular exercise. A daily walk or regular stair climbing fits well with everyday life and may be more likely to be adhered to on a regular basis than a series of exercises that the patient sees as bearing little relation to their normal activities.

Rehabilitation may be unfamiliar territory for the primary care team. When advising about exercise there can be understandable concerns if the patient also suffers from ischaemic heart disease. It may be better, therefore, to start with an 'uncomplicated' patient and to keep advice simple and practical. Giving your patients the following cycle of exercises can be a useful starting point.

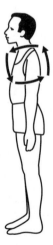

1 Shoulder shrugging.
Circle your shoulder forwards, down, backwards and up. Keep the timing constant, allowing two full seconds per circle and relax throughout. Continue for 30 seconds. Repeat the exercise three times with short rests in between.

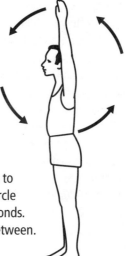

2 Full arm circling.

One arm at a time, pass your arm as near as possible to
the side of your head; move your arm in as large a circle
as possible (10 seconds per circle). Repeat for 40 seconds.
Repeat the exercise three times with short rests in between.
Do the same now with the other arm.

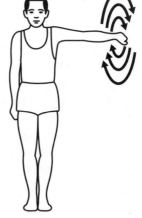

3 Increasing arm circles.

Hold one arm away from your body at shoulder
height. Progressively increase the size of the circle
for a count of six circles in 10 seconds, then
decrease it over a further count of six. Repeat for
40 seconds. Do the same now with the other arm.

4 Abdominal exercises.

Sitting in chair, tighten your abdominal muscles, hold for a count of four
and then release the muscles over four seconds to the starting position.
Repeat continuously for 30 seconds. Do the procedure three times with
short rests in between.

*(Exercise instructions and drawings on pages 120–123 reproduced
by permission of the National Respiratory Training Centre.)*

5 Wall press-ups.
Stand with your feet a full arm's length away from the wall, place your hands on wall and bend at the elbows until your nose touches the wall. Push your arms straight again, allowing eight seconds from start to completion. Repeat for 40 seconds continuously to a total of five repetitions. Repeat the procedure three times with short rests in between.

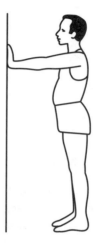 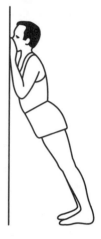

6 Sitting to standing.
Using an ordinary chair, sit, stand and sit, allowing 10 seconds from start to completion. Repeat continuously for 40 seconds to a total of five repetitions. Do the exercise three times with short rests in between.

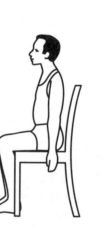 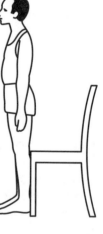

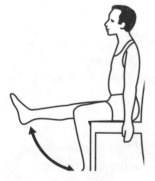

7 Quadriceps exercise.
Sitting on an ordinary chair, straighten your right knee and tense your thigh muscles; hold for a count of four, then relax gradually over a further four seconds. Do this a total of five repetitions over 40 seconds. Repeat the exercise three times with short rest periods in between. Do the same now with your left leg.

8 Calf exercises.
Holding onto the back of
a chair, go up on your toes
and then back, taking
8–10 seconds to complete
procedure. Repeat this
continuously for
40 seconds.

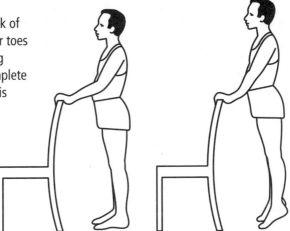

9 Walking on the spot.
Holding onto the back of a chair, allow one knee to bend, keeping your toes
on the ground. Bend the other knee while straightening the first knee,
allowing four seconds for the complete procedure. Repeat this bending
and straightening of your knees
(i.e. walking on the spot),
keeping your toes on the
ground, continuously for
40 seconds – a total of
10 times. Repeat the
exercise three times
with short rest
periods in
between.

10 Step-ups.
Step up with your right foot onto step then bring up your left foot. Step
down with your right foot and then your left foot. Allow four seconds for
the complete procedure and repeat continuously for 40 seconds – a total of
10 times. Repeat the exercise three times with short rest periods between.

The family focus of primary care and its ability to provide long-term follow-up and care make it an ideal setting for the education, follow-up and encouragement of COPD patients and their families.

Finally, when you are encouraging someone to exercise, the type is perhaps less important than its regularity. It is important not to deter patients with too rigid or complicated an exercise regimen. The essence is to encourage, to reassure that they will do themselves no harm and, perhaps most important of all, to persuade them that they are worth the effort.

Further reading

GOLDSTEIN RS, GORT EH, STUBBING D, AVENDANO MA, GUYATT GH (1994) Randomised controlled trial of respiratory rehabilitation. *Lancet* **344**: 1394–7

GRIFFITHS TL, PHILLIPS CJ, DAVIES S, BURR ML, CAMPBELL IA (2001) Cost effectiveness of an outpatient multidisciplinary pulmonary rehabilitation programme. *Thorax* **56**: 779–84

HODGKIN JE (1990) Pulmonary rehabilitation. *Clinics in Chest Medicine* **11**: 447–60

LACASSE Y, WONG E, GUYATT GH et al. (1996) Meta-analysis of respiratory rehabilitation in chronic obstructive pulmonary disease. *Lancet* **348**: 1115–89

MORGAN M, SINGH S (1997) *Practical Pulmonary Rehabilitation.* Chapman and Hall Medical, London.

NIEDERMAN MS, CLEMENTE PH, FEIN AM et al. (1991) Benefits of a multidisciplinary pulmonary rehabilitation program. Improvements are independent of lung function. *Chest* **99**: 798–804

REISS AL, KAPLAN RM, LIMBERG TM, PREWITT LM (1995) Effects of pulmonary rehabilitation on physiologic and psychosocial outcomes in patients with chronic obstructive pulmonary disease. *Annals of Internal Medicine* **122**: 823–32

SINGH SJ, MORGAN MDL, HARDMAN AE et al. (1994) Comparison of oxygen uptake during a conventional treadmill test and the shuttle walking test in chronic airflow limitation. *European Respiratory Journal* **7**: 2016–20

TOSHIMA MT, KAPLAN RM, REISS AL (1990) Experimental evaluation of rehabilitation in chronic obstructive pulmonary disease: short-term effects on exercise endurance and health status. *Health Psychology* **93**: 237–52

WIJKSTRA PJ, TEN VERGERT EM, VAN ALTENA R et al. (1990) Long term benefits of rehabilitation at home on quality of life and exercise tolerance in patients with chronic obstructive pulmonary disease. *Thorax* **50**: 824–8

Useful address

Breathe Easy Club
British Lung Foundation
73–75 Goswell Road
London EC1V 7ER
Tel: 020 7688 5555
Fax: 020 7688 5556
Website: www.lunguk.org

Other forms of therapy

Main points

Oxygen

1 Long-term oxygen therapy (LTOT) improves breathlessness and survival in severe COPD.

2 To be effective, LTOT must be administered for at least 15
hours per day.

3 The most cost-effective way of administering oxygen over
long periods is by oxygen concentrator. This also allows
the patient much greater mobility around the home while
still receiving oxygen.

4 Ambulatory oxygen is available from small cylinders but
these last only a few hours and are not very practical.

5 Patients with severe COPD need specialist advice before
flying or travelling to high altitude.

Surgery

1 The surgical removal of large bullae may significantly
improve lung function and symptoms.

2 Surgery to reduce lung volume is gaining in popularity
but should be performed only in specialist centres and
with careful patient selection. It has an operative mortality
of 1–3% but can produce good clinical improvements.

3 Lung transplants are usually performed on younger
patients (below 50 years) with alpha-1 antitrypsin
deficiency emphysema.

Vaccination

1 Vaccination annually against influenza is recommended.

2 The Department of Health recommends pneumococcal vaccination for patients with COPD.

Nutrition

1 Diets rich in antioxidants (e.g. fresh fruit and vegetables) may help to slow the progress of COPD.

2 Obese patients should be vigorously encouraged to lose weight, which will reduce breathlessness and improve mobility.

3 Many patients with advanced emphysema are under-weight and have extensive muscle wasting. The mechanism is not certain but inflammatory cytokines may have a role.

4 Patients with muscle wasting need advice on an appropriate diet.

5 The life expectancy is worse for COPD patients who are underweight and have muscle wasting.

Oxygen therapy

Patients with severe COPD who are in chronic respiratory failure benefit from oxygen, but it has to be given over long periods every day. The aims of long-term oxygen therapy (LTOT) are thus quite different from the short-term use of oxygen in hospital for patients with acute exacerbations.

At sea level the atmosphere contains around 21% oxygen. LTOT aims to increase the concentration of oxygen in inhaled air to around 30%. This level generally provides the best tissue oxygenation without increasing the arterial carbon dioxide and worsening the respiratory failure. The results of two placebo-controlled trials of LTOT revealed:

■ improved survival,

■ reduced polycythaemia,

■ no progression of pulmonary hypertension,

■ slightly improved health status.

The first of these trials, conducted by the Medical Research Council (MRC), showed that 15 hours of oxygen per day increased five-year survival from 25% to 41%. The second trial – the Nocturnal Oxygen Therapy Trial (NOTT) – demonstrated that continuous oxygen (mean use of 17.7 hours per day) was beneficial, but that use for only 12 hours per day conferred no benefit.

A further study of patients using 15 hours of oxygen per day showed that, although five-year survival was 62%, this had dropped to only 26% at ten years. Why some patients do better than others is incompletely understood. Generally, the patients who obtained most benefit from LTOT had:

■ a higher $Paco_2$,

■ a higher packed cell volume (haematocrit),

■ a higher pulmonary pressure,

■ a lower FVC.

A good prognostic indicator was a fall in pulmonary artery pressure of more than 5mmHg over 24 hours when oxygen was given.

The clinical benefits of LTOT, apart from increased life expectancy, are an increase in exercise tolerance and reduced breathlessness. Whether LTOT improves health status is debatable. A striking finding in patients being considered for LTOT is the very high level of emotional and mood disturbance. These patients have severe disease: depression is thus very common and low self-esteem almost universal. Whilst the NOTT study did not show any change in health status on oxygen, the results from other studies have indicated improvement in mood and depression indices, well-being and breathlessness scores, exercise tolerance and sleep patterns. Generally, physicians with extensive experience of LTOT are favourably impressed with the improvements in quality of life that these patients can achieve.

Who should receive LTOT?

In general, patients considered for LTOT:

- have severe COPD,

- are hypoxic,

- have evidence of right ventricular strain and peripheral oedema.

It is important that patients are assessed by a respiratory physician. Measurements of lung function and arterial blood gases are needed. If the criteria outlined below are met, the patient needs a trial of oxygen in hospital with further measurement of blood gases to determine what concentration of oxygen is required to correct the hypoxia without causing an undue increase in the level of carbon dioxide. It is essential that arterial blood gases for assessment for LTOT are taken when the patient has been clinically stable for at least a month. Drug therapy should be optimised; steroid trials should have been performed and the possibility of further benefit from increased bronchodilator doses or improved delivery systems investigated. Patients *must* have stopped smoking: smoking in the presence of oxygen constitutes an explosive hazard, and there is evidence that LTOT has no benefit for patients who continue to smoke.

Although the decision to refer a patient for oxygen therapy is best made on clinical grounds together with the spirometry, pulse oximetry may be a useful screening tool in general practice. If the oxygen saturation is less than 92% when the patient is stable, referral for blood gases and further investigation is likely to be needed. NICE recommends that oxygen saturation be routinely measured in patients whose FEV_1 is less than 50% predicted.

Clinical criteria for LTOT

The following are the recommendations from the Royal College of Physicians of London Clinical Guidelines 1999.

- Patients must be assessed when clinically stable for at least one month.

- They must have been optimally medically managed prior to assessment.

- The Pao_2 should be less than 7.3 kPa or 55mmHg when breathing air. The level of the carbon dioxide tension can be normal or elevated and does not influence the need for LTOT prescription (evidence A).

- LTOT can be prescribed when the Pao_2 is between 7.3 and 8.0kPa together with the presence of one of the following:

  - secondary polycythaemia or nocturnal hypoxaemia (defined as Sao_2 below 90% for at least 30% of the night),

  - peripheral oedema,

  - evidence of pulmonary hypertension (evidence B).

- LTOT is not recommended for a Pao_2 above 8kPa (evidence A).

- LTOT can be used for palliation of dyspnoea in disabling dyspnoea of terminal disease (evidence B).

- In the absence of definitive evidence, it would seem inappropriate to prescribe LTOT to patients unwilling to stop smoking.

Oxygen should correct the blood gases to an arterial oxygen tension (Pao_2) greater than 8kPa, without causing a rise in arterial carbon dioxide ($Paco_2$) that significantly increases the level of respiratory failure.

Oxygen concentrators

In England, Wales and Northern Ireland the patient's GP will be asked to prescribe an oxygen concentrator. In Scotland, concentrators are prescribed by the respiratory physician. Changes to oxygen prescribing are due to come into force in 2005. This will allow the use of all available oxygen-delivery systems: portable oxygen cylinders, liquid oxygen, conservation devices and ambulatory oxygen systems. Patients will be assessed for the most suitable system and supplied by the oxygen company with the franchise to the regional health authority. This should improve the current somewhat haphazard prescription of oxygen and allow the most cost-effective and suitable devices to be made available to patients.

To confer any benefit, LTOT must be used for at least 15 hours per day. This is best achieved using an oxygen concentrator with nasal prongs, at a flow rate of either 2 or 4 litres per minute. The flow rate is determined during the hospital trial and must be stipulated on the prescription for the concentrator. The concentrator is currently prescribed on a standard FP10 form, which is given to the patient. It should contain the following information:

- oxygen concentrator,

- flow rate in litres per minute,

- number of hours per day it should be used,

- back-up oxygen cylinder (if required).

Information on the regional suppliers of concentrators in the UK can be found in the *British National Formulary* (*BNF*). The regional supplier will deliver and install the concentrator and maintain it regularly. The patient is regularly supplied with replacement nasal prongs and tubing. The concentrator contains a meter for recording the number of hours it has been used. This allows the electricity costs to be reimbursed direct to the patient and compliance to be assessed. All regional oxygen supply companies have a 24-hour call-out service in case the concentrator breaks down.

Follow-up blood gas measurement should be performed after six months of treatment. Increasingly, the specialist respiratory nurse at the local chest unit provides regular follow-up and gives the patient and their carers valuable psychological and social support.

Patients using concentrators occasionally have problems with drying of the nasal mucosa and soreness from the nasal prongs. A humidifier can be added into the system but great care is needed with its maintenance to prevent infection. Water-based creams such as E45 around the nostrils may reduce soreness. Using nasal prongs can also cause soreness around the ears and across the cheeks, so the oxygen tubing may need to be padded.

Cost/benefit

The use of domestic size oxygen cylinders (size F) for 15 hours per day costs around £6,500 per year. The cost of a concentrator is considerably less at £1,500, plus about £80 per month for maintenance and £20 per month for electricity, the cost of which is refunded to the patient. The major expense of the concentrator is the installation. Concentrators are very much more convenient for the patient to use and enable greater mobility around the home. A size F cylinder needs to be changed every 11 hours or so, so spare cylinders must be ordered, delivered and stored. It is not possible to fit long lengths of tubing to a cylinder and the patient is effectively 'chained' to the oxygen source. Any benefits in improved exercise tolerance are therefore likely to be undermined. In contrast, up to 50 metres of tubing can be attached to a concentrator, allowing the patient a considerable degree of mobility around the home.

LTOT prolongs life and has some benefits in health status. A French survey of 13,500 patients using LTOT found that 55% of them were able to wash unaided. However, 25% never left their homes and 25% never went on holiday. It is possible that portable oxygen systems might improve this situation.

Ambulatory oxygen therapy

The Royal College of Physicians Guidelines give the following indications for ambulatory oxygen therapy.

- It can be prescribed for inpatients on LTOT who are mobile and need to or can leave the home on a regular basis. The type of portable device will depend on the patient's mobility (evidence B).

- Patients without chronic hypoxaemia and LTOT should be considered for ambulatory oxygen if they show evidence of:

  - exercise oxygen desaturation,

  - improvement in exercise capacity and/or dyspnoea with ambulatory oxygen therapy and the motivation to use the ambulatory oxygen outside the house.

Assessment for ambulatory oxygen

Ambulatory oxygen should be prescribed only after appropriate assessment by a hospital respiratory specialist. The purpose of such assessment is:

- to examine the extent of desaturation and improvement in exercise capacity with supplemental oxygen,

- to evaluate the oxygen flow rate that is required to correct exercise desaturation, aiming to keep the Sao_2 above 90%,

■ to determine the type of ambulatory equipment that is
  required.

Equipment

Although portable oxygen improves exercise tolerance and lessens
breathlessness, encouraging patients to leave their homes and lead a
fuller life, it is used infrequently in the UK. This is caused in part by
the inability to prescribe anything other than small, portable PD,
DD and CD cylinders that provide only two hours of oxygen at 2
litres per minute. Other equipment should be made available on the
drug tariff, with the proposed changes to oxygen prescribing due to
take effect in 2005.

Equipment that is not available for prescription includes oxygen-
conserving devices which target oxygen delivery to specific parts of
the respiratory cycle (only during inspiration) and the more expensive liquid oxygen which can last as long as eight hours at 2 litres per
minute. Such systems are filled from a reservoir kept at the patient's
home, which needs to be regularly topped up as the liquid oxygen
evaporates.

Occasional oxygen use by cylinder

Many patients are prescribed oxygen to be used as required when
breathless, or to enable them to perform activities around the house
more easily. There have been no clinical studies of this role of oxygen
but, anecdotally, patients often find it beneficial. There are no recommendations for such prescribing in the BTS Guidelines. Patients
prescribed oxygen for use in this way might also fit the criteria for
LTOT, and consideration should be given for specialist assessment.

The following are the indications from the RCP Guidelines.

■ Despite extensive prescription of oxygen for short-burst
  use, there is no adequate evidence available for firm
  recommendations.

■ Short-burst oxygen should be considered for episodic
  breathlessness not relieved by other treatments in patients
  with severe COPD or for palliative care.

■ It should be prescribed only if an improvement in
  breathlessness and/or exercise tolerance can be documented.

Travel and flying, and scuba diving

Patients with severe COPD will often require advice about travel, particularly if flying is involved. Aircraft cabin pressures are equivalent to 5000–8000 feet above sea level, which reduces the ambient oxygen pressure to 15–18kPa. In a healthy individual this will reduce mean arterial oxygen from 12kPa to 8.7kPa, with a relatively insignificant drop in oxygen saturation from 96% to 90%. In patients with severe lung disease and hypoxia this reduction in ambient oxygen pressure is likely to cause a potentially hazardous drop in arterial oxygen levels unless they are given supplemental oxygen during the flight.

Other problems may include expansion of emphysematous bullae and abdominal gases resulting in compression of functioning lung. Cabin humidity is reduced on long flights, resulting in potential drying of bronchial secretions.

It has been suggested that, for a patient to be safe to fly:

- the FEV_1 should be in excess of 25% predicted,

- the Sao_2 should be greater than 92%,

- the pre-flight Pao_2 should be greater than 9.3kPa or 70mmHg,

- there should be no hypercapnia.

Airlines often use the yardstick of the person being unable to walk without dyspnoea for more than 50 yards as an indicator for the need of further assessment.

Patients should be encouraged to see a doctor well before they intend to travel so that appropriate tests can be arranged. Airlines need to be approached well in advance and they often require GPs to fill in appropriate data, which a hospital assessment can provide. The airline will usually ask if a flow rate of 2 or 4 litres per minute should be provided.

Oxygen can be arranged on most scheduled flights by prior arrangement, but the cost can vary from nothing at all to £100 per flight, depending on the airline.

Patients with recent pneumothorax or emphysematous bullae may also be at increased risk of spontaneous pneumothorax while flying. Travel by land or sea is usually less of a problem.

If there is any doubt about the advisability of air travel, patients should be referred for assessment by a respiratory physician. Some centres can perform a hypoxic challenge by giving patients air with reduced oxygen levels by cylinder in order to assess their response to the reduced oxygen levels they are likely to experience during a flight.

Scuba diving is not recommended for people with COPD.

Surgery

Treatment of emphysematous bullae

A small proportion of COPD patients may develop large cyst-like spaces – bullae – in the lung. These tend to compress the more normal areas of lung, thus reducing their ability to function efficiently. Large bullae can form in relatively normal lung or with any degree of emphysema. It is not clear how bullae originate but it is most likely that an area of local lung degeneration acts as the focus for an enlarging space. Surgery in such cases can significantly improve symptoms and function.

The symptoms produced by bullae are similar to those from the associated underlying emphysema. They can, however, usually be readily detected on a routine chest x-ray. Rarely, they can present as a pneumothorax. Before surgery is considered, there must be careful specialist physiological assessment and anatomical imaging of the bullae and surrounding lung with CT scanning. The best results are usually obtained in younger patients with large bullae and lesser degrees of airflow obstruction. The degree of emphysema in the surrounding lung is an important determinant of the success of this procedure.

There are a number of surgical approaches, ranging from thoracotomy to a laser technique via a thoracoscope. The aim is to obliterate the abnormal space and restore the elastic integrity of the lung, allowing the compressed areas of the lung to re-expand. Benefits from the surgery are usually felt almost immediately, and the improvement in lung function and symptoms seems to be maintained. Deterioration after the surgery seems to follow the standard course for a patient with emphysema. Operative mortality is low and should decrease further as the preoperative assessment procedures to screen out unsuitable patients improve.

Surgery to reduce lung volume

Lung volume reduction surgery is a relatively new technique. It was developed in the USA but is gaining in popularity in the UK. The operation is performed through a sternal split and involves one or both lungs. The aim is to remove 20–30% of the most distended emphysematous parts of the lungs. The lungs are then stapled and sutured to prevent air leaks. Complications are not uncommon, particularly relating to air leaks. Operative mortality is, at present, 1–3% depending on the centre. Careful preoperative assessment seems to be the key to success.

Lung volume reduction particularly reduces residual volume, improving vital capacity by 20–40%. FEV_1 can increase by between 20% and 80%, and the six-minute walking distance may improve by 30%. Longer term follow-up shows that the peak effect seems to occur at six to eight months following surgery, after which there is a slow decline. However, after two years most patients will still have better lung function than they had before the surgery.

This surgical technique is still in its infancy and many more carefully controlled studies are needed to fully evaluate its usefulness.

An innovative non-invasive technique is currently being developed. It involves the insertion of a one-way valve via a bronchoscope into the airway leading to the worse-affected area of lung. The valve allows air to escape from the lung but will not allow air in. Over a period of a few days the area of lung supplied by that airway collapses, allowing re-expansion of the remaining lung.

Lung transplant

Single lung transplant is the favoured option for emphysema, although double lung transplant procedures can be performed. The operation is generally straightforward and the results are deemed to be excellent. FEV_1 is usually restored to 50% of the predicted value. Lung transplantation is usually offered only to patients under 50 years of age, so the procedure is a likely option for alpha-1 antitrypsin deficiency emphysema, which presents in this young age group. Generally it is considered only for patients with a life expectancy of less than 18 months. UK survival figures are 60% at three years.

The main drawbacks are related to tissue rejection and immunosuppressant therapy. A late and serious complication is the development of obliterative bronchiolitis, which occurs in 30% of patients surviving five years. Unfortunately, this widespread inflammatory fibrotic condition of the small airways is frequently fatal at between six and twelve months.

Vaccinations

Influenza

Vaccination against influenza is recommended for all elderly patients, and has reduced mortality by 70% in this group. It is also indicated for people with a range of chronic diseases, including COPD, and for anyone with decreased immunity. There have been no trials of its efficacy specifically in COPD but, by inference from the data relating to elderly people, there ought to be benefits from regular annual vaccination.

Pneumococcus

Streptococcus pneumoniae is the commonest cause of community-acquired pneumonia. Pneumococcal infection is more common in adults over 50 years; in people over 65 years the risk of infection increases by two- to fivefold. The Department of Health includes COPD patients in its at-risk groups for pneumococcal vaccination. Immunisation should be with the polyvalent vaccine, which is a single injection. Immunocompromised or splenectomised patients should be given booster injections every five years.

There are no controlled studies of the effectiveness of this vaccine in COPD, although an evaluation from the USA concluded that the vaccination of people over 65 years is cost saving.

Nutrition

There is some epidemiological evidence suggesting that diets rich in fresh fruit and vegetables are beneficial in slowing the progression of COPD. Such diets are also, of course, valuable in reducing the risk of coronary artery disease and some cancers. It is thought that the high levels of antioxidants in vitamins C and E have a protective effect on lung tissue. However, a study with vitamin E supplements failed to find any significant benefit compared with a placebo. It is also thought that some natural fish oils may protect the lungs through antioxidant enhancement, but scientific evidence for this is lacking.

Obesity

COPD patients who are overweight are likely to have greater impairment of activity and will experience a greater degree of breathlessness than patients of a normal weight. This in turn causes them to lead a more sedentary existence and have a worsened quality of life. You should encourage overweight patients to lose weight as well as to get regular exercise. (See also Chapter 8.)

Malnutrition and muscle wasting

A low body mass index (BMI) and loss of lean muscle mass are common in COPD, especially when emphysema is the predominant pathological problem. Weight loss is a poor prognostic sign and a low BMI increases the risk of death from COPD.

The cause of weight loss in emphysema is complex and poorly understood. It used to be thought that the chronically increased work of breathing, coupled with difficulties in shopping, preparing food and eating when constantly breathless, caused a negative energy balance and, thus, weight loss. This is now thought not to be the sole cause as, in addition to weight loss, most people with COPD have peripheral muscle weakness linked to loss of muscle mass. It has been discovered that there are systemic inflammatory processes and changes in muscle metabolism in these patients.

Raised levels of certain cytokines, including interleukin 8 (IL-8) and tumour necrosis factor alpha (TNF-α), have been found, and these seem likely to have an important role in causing loss of muscle mass. Increased levels of cytokines may be a response to low levels of oxygen in the tissues (tissue hypoxia), resulting from the destruction of alveoli. This might help to explain why weight loss occurs in some patients with comparatively minor FEV_1 impairment and why patients with chronic bronchitis do not seem to have comparable tissue hypoxia and weight loss.

It should be remembered that loss of muscle mass is also a consequence of the muscle deconditioning that occurs from lack of activity.

It is possible – though difficult – to treat and partially reverse this weight loss. Increased exercise, particularly through a programme of pulmonary rehabilitation, coupled with nutritional supplements and, rarely, anabolic steroids have increased both weight and muscle mass. This may result in a small increase in survival rate for patients who gain weight. Non-steroidal anti-inflammatory drugs (NSAIDs) have been used to block the action of the cytokines that may be involved in causing weight loss in patients with terminal cancer, but this does not seem to have been tried in COPD.

Breathlessness can make the very act of eating tiring. Eating can also induce greater breathlessness. Practical advice to patients includes eating small but frequent high-calorie meals. Fish is more digestible than meat and requires less effort to chew. Pureed vegetables and soups also require less effort to consume. Referral to a dietician may be helpful for some patients.

Exercise

Exercise is an important part of the management of COPD, and is discussed in detail in Chapter 8. Regular exercise is helpful both physically and psychologically, and encourages patients to lead a more normal social life. Encourage patients to regularly walk to the point of breathlessness. Explain that regular walking, pushing themselves a little further each day, will help improve physical fitness. They need reassurance that breathlessness in these circumstances will do no harm to their heart or lungs and is, in fact, positively beneficial. Repeating these positive messages at follow-up visits is helpful.

Social and psychological issues

Many patients with more severe COPD are clinically anxious or depressed. They may feel embarrassed by their breathlessness or inability to exercise, and therefore may tend not to go out and socialise. They may feel guilty about their inability to perform jobs around the house and garden. Impaired activity levels affect both the patient and their partner, family and carers, and can reduce their ability to socialise, take holidays and enjoy a normal life.

Depression should be treated with standard forms of therapy where indicated. Care should be taken, however, not to prescribe medication that might depress the respiratory drive. Small amounts of alcohol are acceptable and, for people with severe COPD who have difficulty sleeping, may be preferable to sleeping pills.

Patients with more severe symptoms should be advised and encouraged to obtain Social Security benefits, which may help to improve their health status. The Citizens Advice Bureaux and the local Department for Work and Pensions can provide information about entitlement to state benefits and how to apply for them.

- The Blue Badge car parking scheme is probably the most practical benefit. Patients whose exercise capability is less than 100 yards on the flat can qualify for a car badge, which allows parking in many restricted areas – enabling easier access to shops, cinema, theatre, beaches and the countryside.

- There are two main disability benefits: the Disability Living Allowance and Attendance Allowance.

  - Disability Living Allowance covers people who need either personal care or help with getting around, or both, because they are ill or disabled. To qualify, they must have needed help for three months and will need it for at least another six months and also be under 65 years of age when this help was first needed. The award depends on how disabled the Department for Work and Pensions reckons the person is.

  - Attendance Allowance is for people 65 and over who need personal care and have needed that help for at least six months.

- Statutory Sick Pay covers employed people who are sick for more than four days; it can be paid for up to 28 weeks. People who are self-employed or unemployed may, if they have paid enough National Insurance contributions, be entitled to Incapacity Benefit. The rate depends on the person's age and how long they have been off work.

- People of working age who have not paid enough National Insurance contributions may qualify for Severe Disablement Allowance if they have not been able to work for at least 28 weeks. They must also have been assessed by the Department for Work and Pensions as being 80% disabled in that time.

- Work-related Industrial Injuries Disablement Benefit is for people who have COPD as a result of exposure to, say, coal dust and this has been established as the cause of their disease.

The Breathe Easy Club of the British Lung Foundation charity provides information and support, and has local groups who meet for social and educational benefits. (For contact details, see the entry in the 'Useful addresses' section.)

Severe breathlessness and palliative care

In end-stage COPD, breathlessness may be so severe that eating and talking become difficult and life is distressing for both patient and carer. Bronchodilators in high doses are the first line of therapy, either by large volume spacer or by nebuliser. Oral prednisolone in doses up to 40mg per day may produce initial improvement, but the benefit is usually small. Oxygen in short bursts from a cylinder is often prescribed.

Palliative therapy

Palliative care has been defined by the World Health Organization as the active, total care of patients whose disease is not responsive to curative treatment. Control of pain, of other symptoms and of psychological, social and spiritual problems is paramount.

There is relatively little information and poor provision of care for this important aspect of the terminal stages of severe COPD. One study compared the needs of patients with COPD and of those with lung cancer and found greater problems in the COPD group. The most common symptoms are extreme breathlessness (95%), pain (68%), fatigue (68%), difficulty sleeping (55%) and thirst (55%).

Organisation of care falls mainly on primary care, with input from hospital respiratory specialists and respiratory nurses, but has a far less effective framework than that for cancer services. There is a great need for an effective strategy and structure.

The NICE guidelines have reviewed the evidence for various therapies to help end-stage breathlessness and have made a number of recommendations.

■ Opiates can be used for the palliation of breathlessness in end-stage COPD unresponsive to other medical therapy.

■ Benzodiazepines, tricyclic antidepressants, major tranquillisers and oxygen should also be used when appropriate.

■ Patients with end-stage COPD should have access to the full range of services offered by multidisciplinary palliative care teams, including admission to a hospice.

A further double-blind study, published since the guideline group met, supports the use of low-dose sustained-release morphine to improve dyspnoea scores and provide a better quality of sleep (Abernethy et al. 2003).

Further reading

Oxygen therapy

COOPER CB, WATERHOUSE J, HOWARD P (1987) Twelve year clinical study of patients with chronic hypoxic cor pulmonale given long-term oxygen therapy. *Thorax* **42**: 105–10

COOPER CB (1995) Domiciliary oxygen therapy. In: Calverley PMA, Pride NB (eds) *Chronic Obstructive Lung Disease.* Chapman and Hall, London; 495–526

DILWORTH JP, HIGGS CMB, JONES PA et al. (1990) Acceptability of oxygen concentrators; the patients' view. *British Journal of General Practice* **40**: 415–17

LAHDENSUO A, OJANEN M, AHONEN A et al. (1989) Psychological effects of continuous oxygen therapy in hypoxic chronic obstructive pulmonary disease patients. *European Respiratory Journal* **2**: 977–80

MEDICAL RESEARCH COUNCIL OXYGEN WORKING PARTY (1981) Report. Long-term domiciliary oxygen therapy in chronic hypoxic cor pulmonale complicating chronic bronchitis and emphysema. *Lancet* **1**: 681–6

NOCTURNAL OXYGEN THERAPY TRIAL GROUP (1980) Continuous or nocturnal oxygen therapy in hypoxic chronic obstructive lung disease. *Annals of Internal Medicine* **93**: 391–8

ROBERTS CM, FRANKLIN J, O'NEILL R et al. (1998) Screening

patients in general practice with COPD for long term
domiciliary oxygen requirement using pulse oximetry.
Respiratory Medicine **92**: 1265–8

ROYAL COLLEGE OF PHYSICIANS OF LONDON (1999) *Domiciliary
Oxygen Therapy Services. Clinical guidelines and advice for
prescribers*. RCP, London

WALTERS MI, EDWARDS PR, WATERHOUSE JC, HOWARD P (1993)
Long term domiciliary oxygen therapy in chronic obstructive
pulmonary disease. *Thorax* **48**: 1170–7

Travel and flying

BRITISH THORACIC SOCIETY STANDARDS OF CARE COMMITTEE.
(2002) Managing passengers with respiratory disease planning
air travel. *Thorax* **57**: 289–304

Surgery

BRENNER M, MCKENNA RJ, GELB AF et al. (1998) Rate of FEV_1
change following lung reduction surgery. *Chest* **113**: 652–9

MCGRAW L (1997) Lung volume reduction surgery: an overview.
Heart and Lung **26**: 131–7

O'BRIEN GM, CRINER GJ (1998) Surgery for severe COPD. Lung
volume reduction and lung transplantation. *Postgraduate
Medical Journal* **103**: 179–94

Nutrition

SCHOLS AMWJ, SLANGEN J, VOLOVICS L et al. (1998) Weight loss
is a reversible factor in the prognosis of chronic obstructive
pulmonary disease. *American Journal of Respiratory and
Critical Care Medicine* **157**: 1791–7

SRIDHAR MK (1995) Why do patients with emphysema lose
weight? *Lancet* **345**: 1190–1

Depression and psychosocial issues

DAVIS CL (2001) Organising the provision of effective palliative
care services for patients with advanced COPD. Chapter 11 in
Wedzicha PI, Miles A (eds) *The Effective Management of
COPD*. Aesculapius Medical Press, London

DUDLEY DL, GLASER EM, JORGENSON BN et al. (1980) Psychosocial concomitants to rehabilitation in obstructive pulmonary
disease. *Chest* **77**: 41

Palliation

ABERNETHY AP, CURROW DC, FIRTH P et al. (2003) Randomised,
double-blind, controlled crossover trial of sustained-release
morphine for the management of refractory dyspnoea. *British
Medical Journal* **327**: 523–6

10

Acute exacerbations and referral to hospital

Main points

1 Exacerbations of symptoms are common, the frequency increasing with more severe levels of COPD. They tend to occur more often in winter.

2 Exacerbations may be infective, characterised by increasing sputum volume, sputum purulence and breathlessness; or they may be related to changes in airflow obstruction, with increased breathlessness, wheeze and cough.

3 Treatment may include:
   – increased bronchodilators,
   – antibiotics,
   – a course of oral corticosteroids for one to two weeks.

4 The decision to manage the exacerbation at home or admit the patient to hospital is based on a list of clinical and social factors summarised in Table 10.1.

5 A prolonged worsening of symptoms should raise the suspicion of other diagnoses (e.g. lung cancer) and lead to further investigation such as chest x-ray and possible referral to hospital.

6 There may be other causes of persistent cough, such as chronic nasal catarrh and postnasal drip. These should be investigated and treated accordingly.

7 The NICE guidelines support a self-management action plan for COPD with early use of antibiotics and oral steroids.

8 The suspicion of respiratory failure in exacerbations should lead to hospital admission and measurement of arterial blood gases.

9 Criteria for referral to a specialist are listed in Table 10.2.

Acute exacerbations of COPD are common and create a large burden on health resources. A UK survey of medical hospital admissions showed that 25% of acute admissions are respiratory, COPD accounting for more than half of these. The average hospital stay was almost 10 days. A recent study in East London has suggested that GP consultations under-estimate the true number of exacerbations by about 50%, the remainder not being reported by patients.

Exacerbations may also cause a marked worsening of symptoms and quality of life, some patients not recovering to baseline levels for up to two months. More frequent exacerbations may be associated with a more rapid decline in lung function and increased mortality.

Defining an exacerbation

Although exacerbations are common, there is no generally accepted definition of an exacerbation of COPD. An International Consensus Group (Rodriguez-Roisin, 2000) defined an exacerbation as:

> a sustained worsening of the patient's condition, from the stable state and beyond normal day-to-day variations, that is acute in onset and necessitates a change in regular medication in a patient with underlying COPD.

Earlier definitions (Anthonisen et al., 1987) have been based on an increase in symptoms of dyspnoea, sputum volume and sputum purulence, with or without symptoms of upper respiratory tract infection.

The new NICE guidelines have defined an exacerbation as a sustained worsening of the patients' symptoms from their usual stable state, which is beyond normal day-to-day variations and is acute in onset. Common symptoms are worsening breathlessness, cough, increased sputum production and change in sputum colour. The change in symptoms often necessitates a change in medication.

Exacerbations become more common with increasing severity of COPD. Once patients start to have acute exacerbations, they will continue to have more. Patients who continue to smoke, according to the US Lung Health Study, are more likely to have more exacerbations and also more likely to encourage long-term colonisation of the airways with *Haemophilus influenzae*. Patients with worse health status scores on the St George's Respiratory Questionnaire tend to have more exacerbations and a greater mortality.

The East London study followed a group of 101 patients with moderate to severe COPD for two and a half years and reported a median rate of 2.4 exacerbations per patient per year. Exacerbations occur more commonly during the winter months. Most of them can be managed in the community but more symptomatic patients, or those whose social circumstances are poor, are likely to need admission to hospital.

Common symptoms of exacerbations are:

- increases in sputum purulence (white sputum becoming yellow or green),

- increases in sputum volume,

- increased breathlessness, wheeze and chest tightness,

- sometimes, fluid retention with ankle swelling.

Exacerbations can be triggered in three ways:

- Infections – both viral and bacterial. According to the East London studies, about 50% of infections are triggered by rhinoviruses and respiratory syncytial viruses, and often start as a cold or upper respiratory infection. However, not all colds lead to exacerbations, and the East London data suggest that only 53% progress to exacerbations. Viral infections tend to cause an exacerbation of longer duration than do bacterial infections. Symptoms usually include an increase in sputum production and a change in sputum colour to yellow or green, and may be accompanied by a fever. Studies by Stockley's group (2000) in Birmingham examined sputum colour during exacerbations and correlated it with bacterial counts and efficacy of antibiotic treatment. Only deep yellow or green sputum is associated with significant pathological bacterial growth, so antibiotics should be reserved for patients with this pattern of sputum production.

- Increases in air pollution.

- A third of exacerbations have no obvious cause but changes occur in lung mechanics and airflow obstruction, such that patients experience greater breathlessness, wheeze and chest tightness but without evidence of infection.

The cause of worsening lung function is frequently not clear. COPD patients often report brief worsening of symptoms on days that are cold, damp or windy but measured lung function on such occasions usually remains unchanged.

Increasing or worsening symptoms may also be caused by other disease processes, and the following should be considered from the history and examination:

■ pneumonia,

■ pneumothorax,

■ pulmonary oedema,

■ pulmonary embolism,

■ lung cancer,

■ upper airway obstruction or foreign body.

Management of the acute exacerbation

Clinical examination during an acute exacerbation is likely to reveal a patient who is breathless, wheezy and coughing, and whose PEF is lower than usual. They may also be cyanosed and have peripheral oedema. A patient who is drowsy, dehydrated or confused is usually in significant respiratory failure and will need urgent admission to hospital. It is helpful to know the patient's usual clinical state so that comparisons can be made. An assessment of the social circumstances and the patient's ability to cope at home are as important as the clinical assessment when making the important decision about whether to manage them at home or to admit them to hospital. The NICE guidelines outlined in Table 10.1 give some pointers.

Natural history of an exacerbation

The East London cohort studies have provided considerable clinical information on the course and outcomes of exacerbations in moderate and severe COPD. The group of 101 patients were followed for two and a half years with daily symptom diary cards and peak flow readings; 34 of them also recorded daily spirometry. Deterioration in symptoms often occurred without change in peak flow. Falls in

Table 10.1 Deciding whether to treat an acute exacerbation at home or in hospital

	Treat at home	*Treat in hospital*
Able to cope at home	Yes	No
Breathlessness	Mild	Severe
General condition	Good	Poor, deteriorating
Level of activity	Good	Poor, confined to bed
Cyanosis	No	Yes
Worsening peripheral oedema	No	Yes
Level of consciousness	Normal	Impaired
Already receiving LTOT	No	Yes
Social circumstances	Good	Living alone/not coping
Acute confusion	No	Yes
Rapid rate of onset	No	Yes
Significant co-morbidity (particularly cardiac and insulin-dependent diabetes)	No	Yes
Also available at hospital		
Changes on the chest x-ray	No	Present
Arterial pH level	> 7.35	< 7.35
Arterial Pao$_2$	> 7kPa	< 7kPa
Local availability of hospital-at-home services	Yes	No

The more referral indicators that are present, the more likely the need for admission to hospital.

lung function were generally small (median fall in peak flow of 6.6 litres/min) and not useful in predicting exacerbations. Larger falls in peak flow were associated with dyspnoea or colds or were related to longer recovery times from the exacerbation.

The median time to recovery of peak flow was six days, and of symptoms seven days. However, at 35 days peak flow had returned to normal in only 75%; at 91 days, 7% had still not returned to their baseline lung function. Prolonged recovery was linked to increased dyspnoea and colds.

In patients with frequent exacerbations there are higher basal levels of inflammatory markers, such as interleukins IL-6 and 8, in the lung. As the severity of COPD increases, there seem to be greater levels of persistent bacterial colonisation of the airways and, accordingly, more inflammatory markers. Each of these is associated with more rapid decline in FEV_1. A recently published longitudinal study from the East London group has shown that, over time, patients experiencing exacerbations have more symptoms of longer duration and have a longer recovery time to baseline.

The effect of exacerbations on quality of life was also assessed. Patients with more frequent exacerbations (more than three per year) had significantly worse quality of life than those with fewer exacerbations. This suggests that exacerbation frequency is an important determinant of health status in COPD and, therefore, an important outcome measure.

The original study of Fletcher and Peto in the 1970s suggested that exacerbations made little difference to the rate of decline in FEV_1 over long periods of time. The East London studies and also the Copenhagen City study challenge this conclusion and infer that exacerbations may accelerate the decline in FEV_1.

Patients with exacerbations have a high rate of readmission to hospital, and a mortality of 20% at 60 days and 47% at one year.

Treatment in the community

Antibiotics

It is common practice to prescribe antibiotics for infective exacerbations of COPD. A meta-analysis of the use of antibiotics compared with a placebo revealed a small but statistically significant benefit in the group treated with antibiotics. The greatest benefit is seen in those with more severe COPD.

The criteria for using antibiotics should include two or more of the following:

- purulent sputum (the most important criterion),
- increased sputum volume,
- increased breathlessness.

The most common pathogen is *Haemophilus influenzae*, with *Streptococcus pneumoniae* and *Moraxella catarrhalis* found less commonly. Occasionally, *Chlamydia pneumoniae* is found. The most appropriate antibiotic should follow local microbiology guidelines but standard antibiotics such as amoxycillin, erythromycin and tetracycline, all for seven days, are normally satisfactory. Sputum culture is not usually indicated.

Bronchodilators

For both infective and non-infective exacerbations, the dose of beta-2 agonist and/or anticholinergic inhaled bronchodilators should be increased, or started four-hourly if the patient is not already taking a bronchodilator. Multiple doses of inhaled bronchodilators are safe and can be administered to very breathless patients via a large volume spacer. It is rare that a nebuliser is needed for acute attacks, as high doses of bronchodilator via the large volume spacer have been shown to be just as effective. The addition of theophyllines is of less certain benefit and the small extra improvements that might be gained must be balanced against potential side-effects.

Oral corticosteroids

Oral steroids were of significant benefit in exacerbations in two recent randomised placebo-controlled trials. Both studies showed a more rapid improvement in lung function and symptoms and a shorter hospital stay in the group treated with steroids. Treatment failures were fewer and the time to the next exacerbation was extended in the steroid group.

Steroids may be helpful in exacerbations not caused by infection, where lung function has deteriorated significantly. They may also be added to antibiotics for an infection accompanied by marked wheeze and breathlessness. A course of prednisolone 30mg per day is given for 7–14 days and is usually then discontinued unless the patient has failed to recover fully.

Patients already on long-term oral steroids should have the dose increased to 30–40mg per day; on recovery the dose should be reduced over several weeks back to the previous baseline level.

Follow-up

Exacerbations treated in the community normally respond well to the therapy outlined above. Patients who fail to respond need further examination and review. An important differential diagnosis to exclude in a patient who is slow in responding is lung cancer. If this is suspected, a chest x-ray should be performed and consideration given to referral to a respiratory specialist.

Follow-up is a good opportunity to assess the patient's clinical state, treatment and social circumstances and also to reiterate messages about smoking, weight loss and exercise.

Recurrent exacerbations

Someone with severe COPD may have many exacerbations in a year. The presence of persistent purulent sputum, perhaps with inspiratory coarse crackles – particularly at the lung bases – may suggest a diagnosis of bronchiectasis.

A study by O'Brien et al. (2002) in Birmingham examined the physiological and radiological (high-resolution CT scan) features of 110 patients presenting to their GP with an acute exacerbation of COPD. There was CT scan evidence of bronchiectasis in 29%, and in 51% radiological emphysema. Only 5% had reversibility levels to suggest asthma. The entry criteria for the study involved sputum production; it is likely that, in a more random selection of COPD patients where irreversible airflow is the main criterion, the prevalence of bronchiectasis would be lower. However, the study serves to underline the heterogeneous nature of COPD and the need to be alert to the possibility of coexisting bronchiectasis. Alternatively, and fairly rarely, patients may have an immune deficiency syndrome or abnormality of cilial function (immotile cilia syndrome).

Persistent nasal catarrh and postnasal drip can cause a productive cough. Treating the nose with decongestants and/or a course of betamethasone and neomycin nose drops, given with the correct technique, may clear the nose and reduce the cough.

Prevention of acute exacerbations

We have seen that exacerbations severely impair quality of life, may speed the rate of decline in lung function, are a major cause of GP consultations and hospital admissions and also are the greatest healthcare burden on the community. Preventing or reducing the severity or duration of an exacerbation is therefore an important but sadly neglected goal in the management of COPD.

Some of the new therapies may lengthen the time between exacerbations, and the role of self-management plans needs to be fully explored and assessed.

- Vaccination against influenza is of proven benefit in reducing illness and mortality. Pneumococcal vaccine ought to be of value but its role in COPD has yet to be confirmed.

- Inhaled steroids reduce the number and rate of exacerbations but only in more moderate to severe COPD. The dose–response effect of this action has not yet been studied.

- Long-acting beta-2 agonists such as salmeterol and formoterol have, in a number of studies, extended the time between exacerbations. The new long-acting anticholinergic, tiotropium, has similar properties.

- The combined long-acting beta-2 agonist/inhaled steroid have an additive effect in reducing the frequency of exacerbations.

- Mucolytic agents such as carbocisteine have, in a meta-analysis, also significantly decreased the frequency of exacerbations.

Self-management

Self-management plans for people with asthma have improved symptoms, reduced exacerbations, achieved higher levels of health status and reduced time off school or work. Patients are given more control of their disease and are instructed to respond early to changes in symptoms. A combination of monitoring of symptoms and of peak flow allows patients to act on any deterioration of asthma rapidly and effectively.

In COPD, self-management plans must be focused on teaching patients to respond appropriately to the first signs of an exacerbation; they are not concerned with the day-to-day variations in symptoms.

A Cochrane review of COPD self-management was published in

2003 by Monninkhof et al. (2003). Twelve studies were examined; they included a variety of interventions and comparisons, all but two of which included elements of lengthy patient-education courses and exercise training/rehabilitation. Only two focused on a simple exacerbation action plan, and the numbers of patients in those studies were too small to analyse separately. The meta-analysis concluded that self-management education had no effect on hospital admissions, emergency room visits, days lost from work or lung function. Patients in the intervention group used antibiotics more commonly and resorted to less rescue medication. Inconclusive results were obtained for symptoms, quality of life and visits to doctors and nurses.

However, a more recent randomised controlled study from Canada (Bourbeau et al. 2003) demonstrated much more positive results. Hospital admissions were reduced by 40%, with a 41% reduction in emergency room visits, and there were significant improvements in the impact scale of the St George's Respiratory Questionnaire. Symptoms did not differ between intervention and control groups.

On the basis of these findings, the NICE guidelines expressed the view that the effects of self-management looked promising but would benefit from more studies focusing on an exacerbation action plan.

NICE recommendations on self-management

Patients at risk of exacerbations should be given self-management advice in terms of an action plan that encourages them to respond promptly to the symptoms of an exacerbation (evidence A).

- Start oral steroids if breathlessness increases and interferes with activities of daily living.

- Start antibiotics if sputum becomes purulent.

- Adjust bronchodilator therapy to control symptoms.

Suitable patents should be prescribed a supply of antibiotics and prednisolone to keep at home for use as part of the self-management strategy. They should be advised to contact a healthcare professional if they do not improve.

Stockley et al. have developed a credit-card-sized sputum colour chart for patients to help them to tell when a significant infection is present – i.e. when the sputum is green. Hopefully, this will be commercially available in the near future to help with patient action plans.

Hospital-at-home schemes for acute exacerbations

There is a growing trend for patients with acute exacerbations of COPD who are admitted to hospital to have an initial assessment and, if they are suitable, to be returned home and managed by regular visits from a specialist respiratory nurse from the hospital.

Patients are examined and undergo investigations such as chest x-ray, oxygen saturation, blood gases and spirometry; enquiries are also made about their social circumstances and mental state. Those who are felt to be affected less severely and are socially suitable are returned home and managed by a respiratory nurse who visits daily until their recovery or will readmit them to hospital if their condition deteriorates. Alternatively, some patients who are admitted to hospital may be suitable for early discharge and nurse-supervised home management.

Controlled studies of hospital-at-home schemes have shown that outcomes such as clinical complications and readmission rates are comparable to those treated in hospital. Patients seem to be very satisfied with being treated at home by a nurse.

Respiratory failure

Respiratory failure is a clinical state characterised by severe hypoxia (Pao_2 less than 7.3kPa), with or without accompanying hypercapnia. The diagnosis is made by measurement of arterial blood gases.

Respiratory failure may accompany exacerbations of COPD. Clinical suspicion of hypoxia includes cyanosis and breathlessness. A raised level of arterial carbon dioxide causes symptoms of central nervous system depression with drowsiness, coma, confusion and mood change. There may also be symptoms of tremor and flap of the hands, muscle jerks and convulsions. The vasodilator effect of raised carbon dioxide results in a bounding pulse, flushed skin and headache, sometimes related to papilloedema. Such patients will always need urgent admission to hospital.

Great care must be taken with oxygen therapy on the way to

hospital. Inspired oxygen of 28% via Venturi mask or 2 litres per minute via nasal cannula is the maximum that is safe in an ambulance or at home. Higher levels of inspired oxygen can remove hypoxic respiratory drive and lead to respiratory arrest.

Treatment of associated conditions

Patients with severe COPD frequently develop pulmonary hypertension and cor pulmonale, usually presenting as peripheral oedema. The addition of diuretics and possibly an ACE inhibitor is indicated in patients with:

- peripheral oedema,
- a raised jugular venous pressure, and
- gallop heart rhythm.

There is no effective therapy for pulmonary hypertension alone but patients with cor pulmonale and right heart failure may benefit from long-term oxygen therapy (LTOT).

Consideration of specialist referral

The indications for specialist referral include:

- to make a diagnosis,
- to perform spirometry,
- to exclude other possible diagnoses such as lung cancer,
- to assess for oxygen therapy or long-term nebuliser treatment,
- to offer special advice to younger patients with alpha-1 antitrypsin deficiency.

The indications for specialist referral as set out in the NICE guidelines are listed in Table 10.2

Table 10.2 Indications for specialist referral

Reason	Purpose
Therapeutic advice	
Suspected severe COPD	Confirm diagnosis and optimise therapy
Onset of cor pulmonale	Confirm diagnosis and optimise therapy
Assessment for oxygen therapy	Optimise therapy and measure blood gases
Assessment for nebuliser therapy	Exclude inappropriate prescriptions
Assessment for oral corticosteroids	Justify need for long-term treatment or to supervise withdrawal
Bullous lung disease	Identify candidates for surgery
A rapid decline in FEV_1	Encourage early intervention
Diagnostic advice	
Aged under 40 years or a family history of alpha-1 antitrypsin deficiency	Identify alpha-1 antitrypsin deficiency; consider therapy and screen family
Uncertain diagnosis	Make a diagnosis
Symptoms disproportionate to lung function deficit	Look for other explanations
Frequent infections	Exclude bronchiectasis

Further reading

ANTHONISEN NR, MANFREDA J, WARREN CPW et al. (1987) Antibiotic therapy in exacerbations of chronic obstructive pulmonary disease. *Annals of Internal Medicine* **106**: 196–204

BOURBEAU J, JULIEN M, MALTAIS F et al. (2003) Reduction of hospital utilization in patients with chronic obstructive pulmonary disease – A disease specific self management intervention. *Archives of Internal Medicine* **163**: 585–91

BURGE S, WEDZICHA JA (2003) COPD exacerbations: definitions and classifications. *European Respiratory Journal* **21** (suppl 21): 46s–53s

DAVIES L, ANGUS RM, CALVERLEY PMA (1999) Oral corticosteroid in patients admitted to hospital with exacerbations of COPD: a prospective randomised trial. *Lancet* **354**: 456–60

DONALDSON GC, SEEMUGAL TAR, PATEL IS et al. (2003) Longitudinal changes in the nature, severity and frequency of COPD exacerbations. *European Respiratory Journal* **22**: 931–6

MONNINKHOF EM, VAN DER VALK P, VAN DER PALEN J et al. (2003) Self-management education for patients with chronic obstructive pulmonary disease: a systematic review. *Thorax* **58**: 394–8

NIEWOEHNER DE, ERBLAND ML, DEUPREE RH et al. (1999) Effect of systemic glucocorticoids on exacerbations of COPD. *New England Medical Journal* **340**: 1941–7

O'BRIEN C, GUEST PJ, HILL SL, STOCKLEY RA (2000) Physiological and radiological characteristics of patients diagnosed with chronic obstructive pulmonary disease in primary care. *Thorax* **55**: 635–42

RODRIGUEZ-ROISIN R (2000) Towards a consensus definition for COPD exacerbations. *Chest* **117**: 398S–401S

SAINT S, BENT S, GRADY D (1995) Antibiotics in COPD: a meta-analysis. *Journal of the American Medical Association* **273**: 957–60

SEEMUNGAL TAR, DONALDSON GC, PAUL EA et al. (1998) Effect of exacerbation on quality of life in patients with COPD. *American Journal of Respiratory and Critical Care Medicine* **157**: 1418–22

SEEMUNGAL TAR, DONALDSON GC, BHOWMIK A et al. (2000) Time course and recovery of exacerbations in patients with COPD. *American Journal of Respiratory and Critical Care Medicine* **161**: 1608–13

STOCKLEY RA, O'BRIEN C, PYE A, HILL SL (2000) Relationship of sputum colour to nature and outpatient management of acute exacerbations of COPD. *Chest* **117**: 1638–45

11 The NICE COPD guidelines 2004 – a summary of the new features

Main points

1 Diagnosis. COPD should be considered in smokers and ex-smokers over 35 years who have one or more of: breathlessness on exertion, chronic cough, regular sputum production, winter bronchitis or wheeze.

2 Smoking cessation is the most important component of COPD managment. All patients should be encouraged to stop, and offered help, at every opportunity.

3 Inhaled therapy. Long-acting bronchodilators should be used to control symptoms and improve exercise capacity in patients who continue to experience problems despite the use of short-acting drugs. Inhaled steroids should be added to long-acting bronchodilators, in order to decrease exacerbation frequency, in patients with FEV_1 less than 50% predicted and who have had two or more exacerbations per year.

4 Pulmonary rehabilitation should be offered to all patients who consider themselves functionally disabled.

5 The frequency of exacerbations should be reduced by appropriate use of inhaled steroids and long-acting bronchodilators and by vaccinations. Self-management action plans should be encouraged.

6 Multidisciplinary teams play a key role in the delivery of care in COPD.

These new guidelines were commissioned by the National Institute for Clinical Excellence (NICE) and were researched and written by the National Collaborative Centre on Chronic Conditions to the highest evidence-based standards. They have the full support of the British Thoracic Society (BTS) and were published in full format with all evidence tables and references in *Thorax*, March 2004. Other

nd patient-orientated versions of the guideline are available
... ... NICE website. The BTS COPD Consortium is producing a
short summary document to be distributed to all primary care and
some secondary care practitioners, and teaching slides on Power-
point will be available, free, to download from the BTS website.

This new chapter does not attempt to summarise the whole
NICE guideline, as many of the latest features are already in the
appropriate chapters and are not significantly different from this
book's previous edition in 2002. The aim is to highlight the new
definitions of COPD, criteria for diagnosis and changes in management in one section, which will allow ready access for the reader.

Definition

COPD is characterised by airflow obstruction. The airflow obstruction is usually progressive, not fully reversible and does not change
markedly over several months. The disease is predominantly caused
by smoking.

- Airflow obstruction is defined by spirometry as a reduced
  FEV_1 of less than 80% of predicted value, plus a reduced
  FEV_1/FVC ratio below 70%.

- Airway obstruction is due to a combination of airway and
  parenchymal lung tissue damage.

- Damage is the result of chronic inflammation that differs
  from that seen in asthma and which is usually the result of
  tobacco smoke.

- Significant airflow obstruction may be present before the
  individual is aware of it.

- COPD produces symptoms, disability and impaired quality
  of life, which may respond to pharmacological and other
  therapies that have limited or no impact on the airflow
  obstruction.

- COPD is the preferred term for patients with airflow
  obstruction who were previously diagnosed as having chronic
  bronchitis or emphysema.

- Other factors, particularly exposure at work, may also
  contribute to the development of COPD.

Making a diagnosis

There is no single diagnostic test for COPD. Making a diagnosis relies on clinical judgement based on a combination of history, age, physical examination and confirmation of the presence of airflow obstruction using spirometry.

The diagnosis of COPD depends crucially on thinking of it in the first place as a possible cause of breathlessness or cough in any smoker or ex-smoker over the age of 35 years. The key symptoms remain:

- exertional breathlessness,

- chronic cough,

- regular sputum production,

- frequent winter bronchitis,

- wheeze.

Spirometry

Spirometry is still essential for demonstrating airflow obstruction to confirm the diagnosis. It should be performed:

- at the time of diagnosis,

- opportunistically, not more often than once per year,

  or

- to reconsider the diagnosis if a patient has an exceptionally good response to treatment.

Reversibility testing

One of the major changes in the new guidelines is the advice on the role of spirometric reversibility testing to bronchodilators and a trial of oral steroids. Whilst spirometry remains essential for confirming the diagnosis of airflow obstruction, **reversibility testing is no longer routinely recommended for all patients.** The correct diagnosis of COPD, and its differentiation from asthma, can usually be made on clinical grounds and, where necessary, by careful assessment of response to treatment.

The reasoning behind this new stance is based on clinical studies and observations. It is now recognised that there are many difficulties with the old approach and that routine spirometric reversibility testing may be unhelpful or misleading because:

■ Repeated FEV_1 measurements can show small spontaneous fluctuations.

■ The results of reversibility tests performed on the same patient on different occasions can be inconsistent and not reproducible.

■ Over-reliance on a single reversibility test may be misleading unless the change in FEV_1 is very large (e.g. greater than 400ml).

■ The definition of what constitutes the magnitude of a significant change is purely arbitrary (and has varied between 10% and 20% in different settings).

■ Response to long-term therapy is not predicted by short-term reversibility testing.

This stance on routine reversibility testing is shared by both the American and the European Respiratory Societies and may well be adopted by GOLD in the near future.

Differentiation between COPD and asthma

COPD and asthma can usually be distinguished on the basis of history in untreated patients presenting for the first time. Assessing response to treatment and using spirometry, peak flow or change in symptoms are all helpful in differentiating between the conditions. In patients in whom there remains uncertainty about the diagnosis, the following may be of benefit in identifying asthma:

■ FEV_1 and FEV_1/FVC ratio return to normal.

■ A very large (> 400ml) response in FEV_1 to either bronchodilator or prednisolone 30mg daily for two weeks.

■ Serial peak expiratory flow (PEF) readings showing significant (20% or greater) diurnal or day-to-day variability.

If patients report a dramatic improvement in symptoms in response to inhaled therapy, whether in the short term or over a more prolonged period of time, the diagnosis of asthma should be considered. Patients in whom the diagnosis remains uncertain should be referred for specialist advice and more detailed investigations. A comparison of the clinical features of COPD and asthma is given in Table 11.1.

Table 11.1 Clinical features differentiating COPD and asthma

	COPD	*Asthma*
Smoker or ex-smoker	Nearly all	Possibly
Symptoms under age 35	Rare	Often
Chronic productive cough	Common	Uncommon
Breathlessness	Persistent and progressive	Variable
Night waking, breathlessness or wheeze	Uncommon	Common
Significant diurnal or day-to-day variability of symptoms	Uncommon	Common

Classification and assessment of disease severity

Traditionally, the severity of COPD has largely been equated with the $FEV_1\%$ predicted value. We now better understand that COPD is a systemic disease that may affect parts of the body other than the lungs and, thus, disability affecting exercise, the activities of daily living and quality of life and mood has a significant effect on the patient. Mild airflow obstruction can be associated with significant disability. A true assessment of severity should therefore include not only spirometry but also other measures such as:

- a measure of breathlessness (MRC dyspnoea scale),
- enquiry as to how COPD is affecting general daily living,
- frequency of exacerbations,
- weight loss (body mass index),
- oxygen saturation with pulse oximeter,
- the presence of cor pulmonale.

The NICE guidelines have produced new levels of gradation of airflow obstruction according to FEV_1% predicted, shown in Table 11.2. These have been selected:

■ to harmonise with new levels in most international guidelines,

■ to reflect the threshold for undertaking various assessments and starting new treatments.

Table 11.2 Severity of airflow obstruction according to FEV1% predicted

Severity	FEV_1
Mild airflow obstruction	50–80 % predicted
Moderate airflow obstruction	30–49% predicted
Severe airflow obstruction	Below 30% predicted

COPD – a multi-system disease

The new guidelines emphasise that COPD not only affects the lungs and breathing but also has other effects such as muscle wasting and fatigue, weight loss, pulmonary hypertension and cor pulmonale, anxiety and depression. Patients with COPD should therefore have access to a wide range of skills delivered from a multidisciplinary team.

In view of the multi-system nature of the disease, the response to various treatments may be reflected not by conventional improvements in FEV_1 but by changes in symptoms and quality of life measures, frequency of exacerbations, increased exercise tolerance and overall well-being.

New recommendations on drug treatment

Since the initial BTS Guidelines, there have been a considerable number of published studies with grade A or B evidence levels that have clarified the role of some of the newer agents now available for symptomatic relief, improvement of quality of life and prevention of exacerbations.

Inhaled bronchodilators

Short-acting bronchodilators, both beta-agonists and anticholinergics, remain as the initial treatment for the relief of breathlessness and exercise limitation.

The effectiveness of such therapy should not be assessed by lung function alone but should include a variety of other measures such as improvement in symptoms, in activities of daily living and in exercise capacity.

Patients who remain symptomatic should have their inhaled treatment intensified to include long-acting bronchodilators (both beta-agonists and anticholinergics) or combined therapy with a short-acting beta-agonist and short-acting anticholinergic.

Long-acting bronchodilators show added benefits over short-acting therapy and should be added in patients who remain symptomatic despite using short-acting bronchodilators or who have two or more exacerbations per year. The benefits of long-acting bronchodilators include a greater effect on symptom control, a significant improvement in quality of life scores and the ability to reduce the frequency of acute exacerbations.

The choice of drug should be determined on the basis of efficacy, side-effects, patient preference and cost effectiveness.

Inhaled corticosteroids

Oral corticosteroid reversibility tests do not predict response to inhaled steroid therapy, and should not be used to determine which patients should be prescribed inhaled steroids (evidence A).

Inhaled corticosteroids should be prescribed for patients with an FEV_1 less than or equal to 50% predicted who have had two or more exacerbations in the last year. The aim of treatment is to reduce exacerbations and slow the rate of decline in health status, and not to slow the rate of decline in lung function (evidence B).

Combination therapy

Combining therapies from different drug classes is recommended to increase clinical benefit (evidence A). This includes combinations of various bronchodilators and long-acting beta-agonists with corticosteroids.

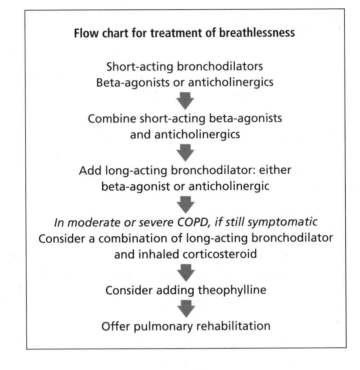

Flow chart for treatment of breathlessness

Short-acting bronchodilators
Beta-agonists or anticholinergics

Combine short-acting beta-agonists
and anticholinergics

Add long-acting bronchodilator: either
beta-agonist or anticholinergic

In moderate or severe COPD, if still symptomatic
Consider a combination of long-acting bronchodilator
and inhaled corticosteroid

Consider adding theophylline

Offer pulmonary rehabilitation

Mucolytic therapy

Mucolytic therapy should be considered in patients with chronic productive cough. The aim of treatment is to reduce frequency of cough and sputum production (evidence B). At present the only agent that can be prescribed in the UK is carbocisteine (Mucodyne).

Pulmonary rehabilitation

The NICE guidelines stress the value to patients of rehabilitation, which should be made available to all appropriate patients.

Rehabilitation is defined as a multidisciplinary programme of care for patients with chronic respiratory impairment that is tailored and designed to optimise each individual's physical and social performance and autonomy. A typical programme incorporates physical training, disease education, and nutritional, psychological and behavioural intervention.

Rehabilitation should be offered to all patients who consider themselves functionally disabled by COPD (usually MRC grade 3 and above). It should be easily accessed by patients in terms of its location and its availability.

Hospital-at-home schemes

Hospital-at-home schemes and assisted early discharge from hospital are recommended as methods to reduce the need for patients with acute exacerbations to be admitted to, or to stay in, hospital.

Treatment of exacerbations

An exacerbation is defined as a sustained worsening of the patient's symptoms from their usual stable state that is beyond normal day-to-day variations and is acute in onset. Common symptoms are worsening breathlessness, cough, increased production of sputum and change in sputum colour. The change in symptoms often necessitates a change in medication.

Pulse oximetry is encouraged in primary care to aid the assessment of clinical severity of an exacerbation.

Primary care management of an exacerbation consists of:

- increase in bronchodilators – consider giving via a nebuliser,
- antibiotics if sputum is purulent,
- prednisolone 30mg daily for 7–14 days.

Patients should be reviewed and their management optimised as appropriate.

Self-management action plans

Patients at risk of exacerbations should be given self-management advice in terms of an action plan that encourages them to respond promptly to the symptoms of an exacerbation (evidence A).

- Start oral steroids if breathlessness increases and interferes with activities of daily living.
- Start antibiotics if sputum becomes purulent.
- Adjust bronchodilator therapy to control symptoms.

Suitable patents should be prescribed a supply of antibiotics and prednisolone to keep at home for use as part of a self-management strategy. They should be advised to contact a healthcare professional if they do not improve.

Palliative care

Patients with end-stage COPD and their family and carers should have access to the full range of services offered by multidisciplinary palliative care teams, including admission to a hospice.

Opiates, benzodiazepines, tricyclic antidepressants, major tranquillisers and oxygen should be used when appropriate for breathlessness in patients with end-stage disease that is unresponsive to other medical therapy.

Assessment of patients with COPD

A summary of the factors to consider when assessing patients with COPD is given in Figure 11.1.

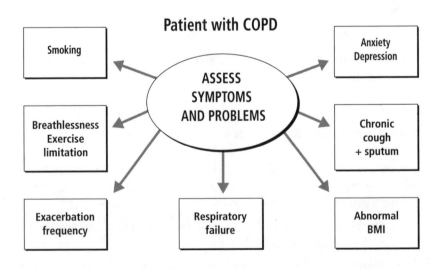

Figure 11.1 Summary of assessment of patients with COPD

Follow-up and monitoring in primary care

Mild to moderate COPD

Patients with mild to moderate COPD should be followed up at least annually. Check on:

- smoking status and desire to quit,
- adequacy of symptom control,
- breathlessness severity,
- exercise tolerance,
- estimate of exacerbation frequency,
- any complications,
- effects of each drug treatment,
- inhaler technique,
- need for referral to specialist and therapy services,
- rehabilitation.

Measurements

- FEV_1 and FVC,
- BMI,
- MRC dyspnoea scale.

Severe COPD

Patients with severe COPD should be followed up at least twice a year, checking on the criteria listed for mild to moderate COPD (above), plus:

- presence of cor pulmonale,
- need for long-term oxygen,
- nutritional status,
- presence of depression,
- need for social services and occupational therapy.

Measurements

- FEV$_1$ and FVC,
- BMI,
- MRC dyspnoea scale,
- Pulse oximetry and oxygen saturation.

12 | The GOLD guidelines

Main points

1 GOLD stands for the Global Initiative for Chronic Obstructive Lung Disease – an attempt to produce guidelines for good COPD management that are applicable throughout the world.

2 The guidelines are evidence-based and compiled by a panel of experts from around the world. They were updated in 2003.

3 GOLD defines COPD as a disease state characterised by airflow limitation that is not fully reversible. The airflow limitation is usually both progressive and associated with an abnormal inflammatory response of the lungs to noxious particles or gases.

4 The classification of severity is based, as are other guidelines, on the level of FEV_1 as a percentage of predicted value plus an FEV_1/FVC ratio below 70%. However, the addition of an at-risk group who have cough or sputum without abnormal lung function helps to highlight the need for early detection of the disease.

5 Spirometry remains the key to making a diagnosis and assessing the severity of disease.

6 Bronchodilator reversibility testing helps to identify patients who may have asthma but is less helpful in measuring clinical response to therapy.

7 GOLD suggests steroid reversibility with a six-week to three-month trial of inhaled corticosteroid rather than two weeks of oral steroids.

8 Smoking cessation is the single most effective way of reducing the development of COPD.

9 Bronchodilators are central to symptomatic treatment.

10 Inhaled steroids have a role in more severe COPD, particularly in patients with more frequent exacerbations.

11 Pulmonary rehabilitation improves both quality of life and exercise capability.

12 Acute exacerbations are managed with increased bronchodilators, antibiotics and oral steroid courses, as indicated by the pattern of symptoms.

What is GOLD?

GOLD is the Global Initiative for Chronic Obstructive Lung Disease – a world-wide strategy for the diagnosis, management and prevention of COPD. The guidelines were produced by an international panel of experts who methodically reviewed the known published scientific literature to produce a set of evidence-based guidance on what is known and, in many cases, not known about the pathogenesis and management of COPD. They were updated in 2003.

The aim of these guidelines is to bring COPD and its care to the attention of governments, public health officials, health care workers and the general public in as many countries around the world as possible, particularly the Third World.

The categories of evidence specified are:

- evidence A: randomised controlled trials – rich body of evidence,

- evidence B: randomised controlled trials – limited body of evidence,

- evidence C: non-randomised trials; observational studies,

- evidence D: panel consensus judgement.

The GOLD definition of COPD

COPD is a disease state characterised by airflow limitation that is not fully reversible. The airflow limitation is usually both progressive and associated with an abnormal inflammatory response of the lungs to noxious particles or gases.

Classification of COPD by severity

The GOLD classification (Table 12.1) has changed to come into line with the new standards set by the American and European Respiratory Societies. However, it retains two groups – 'At risk' and 'Very severe' – that do not appear in other guidelines. The ratio of FEV_1/FVC less than 70% remains the main marker for airflow obstruction but the 'Mild' classification in the updated guideline continues to use an FEV_1% predicted greater than 80% with or without cough or sputum production. This differs from the 'Mild' classification in the old BTS and the NICE guidelines where 'Mild' is assessed by an FEV_1% predicted of less than 80%.

'Very severe' is an FEV_1 less than 30% predicted or can be less than 50% predicted in the presence of respiratory failure. These variations make it less useful for primary care, particularly when coding severity on a computer database.

The Stage 0 – 'At risk' – group helps to highlight patients who

Table 12.1 The GOLD classification of COPD

Stage	Characteristics
At risk	Normal spirometry Chronic cough or sputum production
Mild COPD	FEV_1/FVC <70% FEV_1 >80% predicted With or without chronic symptoms (cough, sputum production)
Moderate COPD	FEV_1/FVC <70% FEV_1 50–80% predicted With or without chronic symptoms
Severe COPD	FEV_1/FVC <70% FEV_1 30–50% predicted With or without chronic symptoms
Very severe COPD	FEV_1/FVC <70% FEV_1 <30 % predicted or FEV_1 <50% plus chronic respiratory failure

have persistent cough or sputum but normal lung function, who may have early disease and may progress to clinical COPD. Identifying patients at this early stage and advising them to stop smoking may prevent the disease from developing.

Goals of management

The goals of COPD management are to:

- prevent disease progression,

- relieve symptoms,

- improve exercise tolerance,

- improve health status,

- prevent and treat complications of COPD,

- prevent and treat exacerbations,

- prevent and minimise side-effects of treatment,

- reduce mortality.

Assessing and monitoring disease

When assessing and monitoring COPD, the following factors should be borne in mind.

- The diagnosis of COPD is based on a history of exposure to risk factors and the presence of airflow limitation that is not fully reversible, with or without the presence of symptoms.

- Patients who have chronic cough and sputum production with a history of exposure to risk factors should be tested for airflow limitation, even if they do not have dyspnoea.

- For the diagnosis and assessment of COPD, spirometry is the gold standard because it is the most reproducible, standardised and objective way of measuring airflow limitation. An FEV_1/FVC <70% and a post-bronchodilator FEV_1 <80% predicted confirm the presence of airflow limitation that is not fully reversible.

■ Health care workers involved in the diagnosis and management of COPD patients should have access to spirometry.

■ Measurement of arterial blood gases should be considered in all patients with an FEV$_1$ <40% predicted or clinical signs suggestive of respiratory or right heart failure.

Main clinical indicators for considering a diagnosis of COPD

The main indicators of COPD are as follows.

■ Chronic cough: intermittent or every day; often present throughout the day but seldom only at night.

■ Chronic sputum production: any pattern can indicate COPD.

■ Dyspnoea that is:

– progressive, worsening with time,

– persistent, being present every day,

– worse with exercise and during respiratory infections.

■ Acute bronchitis – repeated episodes.

■ History of exposure to risk factors, especially tobacco smoke; also to occupational dusts and chemicals, and perhaps smoke from home cooking and heating fuel. Biomass fuels (e.g. charcoal) used for cooking and heating in Third World countries seem to pose a particular risk.

Physical examination Although a physical examination is important, it is rarely diagnostic and has low sensitivity.

Bronchodilator reversibility testing Usually performed only once, at the time of first presentation, bronchodilator reversibility testing is helpful to exclude a diagnosis of asthma, to assess best lung function for prognosis and to help in deciding on treatment. Patients who do not respond significantly to a short-acting bronchodilator test may nevertheless benefit symptomatically from long-term treatment.

Steroid reversibility testing This is the simplest and safest way to identify patients most likely to respond to long-term inhaled steroids. They are given a six-week to three-month trial of inhaled steroids using as criteria for a positive response a 200ml and 15% increase in FEV_1 above baseline.

Chest x-ray A chest x-ray is seldom diagnostic but is valuable in excluding other possible diagnoses.

Alpha-1 antitrypsin screening Perform this in patients under 45 years and/or with a strong family history of COPD.

Reducing risk factors

Although COPD cannot be cured, steps can be taken to reduce the risk factors.

- Smoking cessation is the single most effective and cost-effective way to reduce the risk of developing COPD or to stop its progression (evidence A)

- Brief advice on stopping smoking is effective (evidence A) and should be offered at every visit to a health care provider.

- Several pharmacological treatments such as nicotine replacement therapy and bupropion are of proven value (evidence A) and can supplement counselling to help people to stop smoking.

- Progression of many occupationally induced respiratory disorders can be reduced or controlled by strategies such as extractors, protective masks and so on to reduce levels of particles or gases in the workplace (evidence B).

- Reducing exposure to the fumes of cooking and heating with better ventilation and changing, where possible, to other suitable fuels.

Managing stable COPD

Over all, the approach to managing stable COPD should be a stepwise increase in treatment according to the severity of the disease. In addition, health education improves patients' skills and their ability to cope with illness and health status. It is also effective in helping them to stop smoking (evidence A).

No existing medication has modified the long-term rate of decline in lung function (evidence A). Drug therapy is therefore used to reduce symptoms and complications.

Bronchodilators

Bronchodilator medication is central to symptomatic management (evidence A). It is given as required or regularly to reduce symptoms. The inhaled route is generally preferred. The principal bronchodilators are beta-2 agonists, anticholinergics, theophyllines or a combination of one or more of these drugs (evidence A). All categories of bronchodilators increase exercise capacity in COPD without necessarily producing significant changes in FEV_1 (evidence A). Long-acting beta-2 agonists are more convenient and have improved patients' health status significantly (evidence B). Combining beta-2 agonists and anticholinergics in people with stable COPD produces greater and more sustained improvements in FEV_1 and health status than either drug alone (evidence A).

Inhaled corticosteroids

Regular treatment with inhaled steroids does not modify the long-term decline in FEV_1. Data from four large studies provide evidence that regular treatment with inhaled corticosteroids can reduce the frequency of exacerbations and improve health status in patients with more symptomatic COPD with an $FEV_1 < 50\%$ predicted plus repeated exacerbations (evidence A).

A combination of corticosteroid and long-acting beta-2 agonist was more effective than the individual components in improving quality of life, symptoms and lung function (evidence A).

The dose–response relationships and long-term safety of inhaled steroids in COPD are not known.

GOLD continues to recommend a trial of six weeks to three months with inhaled steroid to identify patients who might benefit and respond from long-term inhaled steroid therapy. It agrees that there is growing evidence to suggest that oral steroid trials are a poor predictor of long-term response to inhaled steroids in COPD.

Oral corticosteroids

Long-term treatment with oral steroids is not recommended for people with COPD (evidence A). There is no evidence of long-term benefit with this treatment and, more important, side-effects such as steroid myopathy may contribute to decreased mobility.

Antibiotics

The use of antibiotics other than to treat infectious exacerbations is not recommended (evidence A). Regular use of antitussives is contraindicated in COPD (evidence D).\

Antioxidants and antitussives

Antioxidant agents, especially *N*-acetyl cysteine, reduce the frequency of exacerbations and might have a role in the treatment of patients with recurrent exacerbations (evidence B). Their use needs fuller evaluation.

Vaccination

Vaccination against influenza can reduce serious illness and death in COPD patients by about 50%, and its annual use is recommended (evidence A). Pneumococcal vaccine is given regularly but evidence to support its general use in COPD is lacking (evidence B).

Rehabilitation

The goals of rehabilitation are to reduce symptoms, improve quality of life and increase physical and emotional participation in everyday activities. All COPD patients benefit from exercise training programmes, improving with respect to both exercise tolerance and symptoms of dyspnoea and fatigue (evidence A). These benefits can be sustained even after a single pulmonary rehabilitation programme.

Oxygen

Long-term administration of oxygen (LTOT) for more than 15 hours per day to patients with chronic respiratory failure increases survival (evidence A) and can also have beneficial effects on their exercise capacity and mental state. The clinical criteria are patients at stage 3 who have:

■ a Pao_2 at or below 7.3kPa (55mmHg) or an Sao_2 at or below 88%, with or without hypercapnia, or

■ a Pao_2 between 7.3 and 8.0kPa or an Sao_2 89%, if there is evidence of pulmonary hypertension, peripheral oedema suggesting right heart failure or polycythaemia (haematocrit/packed cell volume > 55%).

Managing exacerbations

COPD is often associated with acute exacerbations. The economic and social burden of exacerbations is extremely high. The triggers are most commonly infection and air pollution but in about one-third the cause cannot be identified (evidence B). The main symptoms of an exacerbation are increasing breathlessness, increasing sputum production, purulent sputum and, often, chest tightness and wheezing. Treatment may be at home or in hospital. Basic therapy includes:

■ Bronchodilators – initiating the use of bronchodilators or increasing their dose and frequency is beneficial in home management (evidence A). In more severe cases, high-dose nebulised therapy can be given where available.

■ Oral corticosteroids are beneficial in the management of acute exacerbations. They shorten recovery time and help to restore lung function more quickly (evidence A). A dose of prednisolone 40mg daily for 10 days is recommended (evidence D).

■ Antibiotics are effective only when patients with worsening dyspnoea and cough also have increased sputum volume and purulence (evidence B). The choice of antibiotic should reflect local patterns of antibiotic sensitivity.

Future research

The GOLD guidelines include suggestions of worthwhile areas for future research. They are extensively referenced.

The full guidelines can be accessed and downloaded from the free website (see website details in the 'Useful addresses' section).

Further reading

PAUWELS R, BUIST AS, CALVERLEY PMA et al. (2001) Global strategy for the diagnosis, management and prevention of COPD. *American Journal of Respiratory and Critical Care Medicine* **163**: 1256–76

13 Drug therapy of the future

Main points

1 Much research is in progress, looking for new treatments for COPD. The most promising therapies are focused on ways to prevent or block inflammatory changes, mediators and proteolytic enzymes.

2 Early studies indicate that the promising new selective phosphodiesterase inhibitor, cilomilast, has good bronchodilator activity and reduces exacerbations of COPD.

3 Antioxidant therapy, either naturally with fruit and vegetables or with specific agents, may help slow the rate of progression of COPD.

One of the problems with writing books is that they are often out of date by the time they are published. This chapter is therefore confined to:

■ therapy that is likely to appear in the next few years and be relevant and available to primary care,

■ active research that is taking place along potentially beneficial lines.

Anti-inflammatory therapies

Increasingly, the design of new drugs is geared towards the pathological changes that are observed in disease processes. Inflammatory changes are found in the airways of people with chronic bronchitis and, to some extent, the terminal airways of patients with emphysema. There are increases in the number of inflammatory cells, such as neutrophils, T-lymphocytes and alveolar macrophages.

Corticosteroids have a modest effect, so other means of blocking the inflammatory process are being explored.

Leukotriene antagonists have been launched recently and have had a beneficial role in asthma. There have, as yet, been no trials of these agents in COPD but it is unlikely that the currently available drugs that block the leukotriene receptors will have a major role. However, leukotriene LTB4 is a potent stimulator of neutrophils, and its levels are increased in the sputum of COPD patients. Trials are currently in progress with selective LTB4 inhibitors, which may be useful in reducing sputum production and cough in COPD.

Phosphodiesterase-4 (PDE4) inhibitors

The phosphodiesterase family of enzymes are important in the normal functioning of various airway cells. In essence, they break down the very important substance cyclic adenosine mono-phosphate (cyclic AMP), which has a pivotal role in causing smooth muscle relaxation, suppresses the activity of many parts of the inflammatory cascade (particularly neutrophils) and has beneficial effects on the activity of pulmonary nerves. Theophyllines have a non-specific effect on blocking the phosphodiesterase enzymes, thus creating higher levels of cyclic AMP. However, they have been of limited clinical success because of their non-specific action and serious side-effects. The new generation of drugs targeting the most important phosphodiesterase, PDE4, should provide a much more clinically beneficial agent with fewer side-effects.

Early trial results on cilomilast, an oral preparation, have shown good bronchodilator actions in COPD with an 11% increase in FEV_1, sustained positive gains in health status and, of considerable interest, a clinically significant reduction of exacerbations over a six-month trial. This agent is unlikely to be licensed in the UK before 2005.

Antiproteases

There is evidence to suggest that one of the major factors in the development of lung damage and emphysema in COPD is over-activity of proteolytic enzymes released from neutrophils and macrophages. The enhanced cellular breakdown may be related to more enzyme release or decreased protective mechanisms, as in alpha-1 antitrypsin deficiency. Neutrophil elastase inhibitors have been developed but are awaiting clinical trials.

Alpha-1 antitrypsin

The genetically inherited homozygous deficiency of the antiprotease protein alpha-1 antitrypsin leads to the development of emphysema in the third decade of life. Various clinical trials have attempted to replace alpha-1 antitrypsin but the results have generally been disappointing. Alpha-1 antitrypsin can be extracted from plasma but the cost is high. A trial in the USA using weekly intravenous alpha-1 antitrypsin failed to halt the decline in lung function. A nebulised formulation – also very expensive – has been tried but, again, improvements are minimal.

Antioxidants

There is good evidence that active oxygen radicals, present in cigarette smoke, play an important role in damaging the lungs in COPD. They are also released by inflammatory cells such as neutrophils and macrophages. The results of a number of studies have suggested that diets high in fresh fruit and vegetables, which contain many antioxidants, may help to prevent or slow the rate of progress of COPD as well as having favourable effects on various cancers, heart disease and bowel disease.

N-Acetyl cysteine

This drug started life as a mucolytic agent (see also 'Mucolytics' in Chapter 11) but had only mild clinical effects on sputum. However, it also has antioxidant properties and a recent Cochrane review has revealed that it does have beneficial actions in COPD. The results of a meta-analysis against placebo showed a 29% reduction in exacerbations, and those in the group receiving treatment had fewer days of illness. There was no difference in lung function or in adverse events between treatments. In a separate, uncontrolled, study there was a reduction in the rate of decline in FEV_1.

N-Acetyl cysteine is not licensed for use in the UK.

Vitamins

Vitamins C and E have been linked with benefits in COPD but better designed trials are needed to establish a true therapeutic effect.

Pulmonary vasodilators

End-stage COPD usually results in pulmonary hypertension secondary to chronic hypoxia. There are no drugs that specifically reduce pulmonary pressure, but the recently developed angiotensin II inhibitor, losartan, reduces pulmonary artery pressure in COPD.

Further reading

BARNES PJ (1998) New therapies for chronic obstructive pulmonary disease. *Thorax* **53**: 137–47.

POOLE PJ, BLACK PN (2001) Oral mucolytic drugs for exacerbations of COPD: systematic review. *British Medical Journal* **322**: 1271–4

Organisation and training needs

Main points

---

1 Structured primary care management may result in:
 – fewer emergency consultations,
 – improved understanding and self-management skills for patients,
 – rational use of medication.

2 Reappraisal of the practice asthma register may reveal patients who have COPD rather than asthma.

3 Spirometry is crucial for the accurate and early detection of COPD.

4 How and where there should be access to spirometry needs to be decided at local level, and depends on local circumstances.

5 Nurses can provide good structured care for COPD patients but the level of their involvement must depend on their training, and GP support is essential.

6 Good communication among the primary health care team is vital.

7 Audit of the outcomes of COPD care is necessary to the continuing development of good standards of care.

8 In the UK, under the General Medical Services contract, payment can be made to GPs who:
 – can produce a register of COPD patients,
 – have patients on the register who have had spirometry performed,
 – have diagnosed new patients using spirometry and reversibility,
 – have recorded the smoking status of COPD patients and given cessation advice to those who are current smokers,

- have checked inhaler technique in COPD patients who are on inhaled therapy in the last 15 months,
- have recorded the FEV_1 of COPD patients in the last 27 months,
- have given influenza vaccine to their COPD patients in the last 15 months.

COPD in primary care is under-diagnosed and under-treated (or over-treated and under-managed). In an average GP list of 2,500 patients there are likely to be 750 smokers (given an average smoking rate of about 30%), of whom 100–150 will have COPD. In areas of social deprivation where smoking rates are higher, the number of COPD patients will be higher. Many of these patients will not be known to their doctor, because they will have mild to moderate disease – so they will be undiagnosed and untreated. On the other hand, many of those whose disease has progressed will be presenting with recurrent chest infections and some will have been misdiagnosed as suffering from asthma – and will be treated for the wrong condition. Those who have severe COPD are likely to be attending hospital and to have been admitted several times with exacerbations of their disease.

Many general practices now offer structured asthma management clinics and it is often the practice nurse who plays a major role. Patients with COPD may have been treated in asthma clinics along asthma management guidelines with ever-increasing doses of expensive asthma therapies. They may have referred themselves, hoping for a new approach to what, too often, is a debilitating disease; or the GP will have referred them, having run out of ideas about what to do for these 'heart sink' patients.

Until recently, there have been no guidelines as to how these patients should be managed, and there has been little training for primary care physicians and nurses. Management tended to be of the 'crisis intervention' variety and there was little understanding of the concepts of proper assessment, diagnosis or long-term management goals for COPD. Patients were frequently given negative advice:

'There is nothing more that I can do for you.'

'I can't give you a new pair of lungs.'

Recently, however, there has been a resurgence of interest in COPD. Guidelines for COPD management have been published by respiratory physician groups around the world. The British version, the BTS Guidelines (published in 1997), and GOLD have helped to renew interest in COPD. Evidence-based guidelines from NICE and, in the UK, the added incentive of payment for providing care for COPD patients under the General Medical Service contract should help to further improve the care these patients receive.

Recent research has shown that, contrary to previously held beliefs, there are interventions that can improve the quality of life of people with COPD. The proper diagnosis and management of this disease in primary care should result in patients being diagnosed earlier and managed better – and will, hopefully, result in fewer of them being referred for specialist care and repeatedly admitted to hospital. Secondary care is more expensive than primary care.

Patients often prefer not to be admitted to hospital and may find that the GP's surgery is more convenient for them. Structured primary care management may result in:

- fewer emergency general practice consultations,

- the patient and their family having a greater understanding of the disease and improved self-management skills, and

- rational and effective use of medication.

Finding the patients

In order to provide effective management, you must first know who your COPD patients are. It is likely that only those patients with more advanced COPD will be known to you and that many people with moderate disease may have been given an incorrect diagnostic label and are being managed inappropriately. A good starting point, therefore, is to re-examine the practice asthma register, looking particularly at patients over 40 years of age with a current or previous smoking history and who are taking asthma medication. A reassessment of each patient's records and reappraisal of how the diagnosis of asthma was reached may reveal those whose history is more in keeping with a diagnosis of COPD than asthma and those in whom an objective, 'water-tight' diagnosis of asthma is lacking. A synopsis of the features of COPD compared with those of asthma is given in Table 14.1.

Table 14.1 A comparison of the features of COPD and asthma

	COPD	*Asthma*
Onset of symptoms	**Aged 40+ years**	Aged +/– 40 years, 'childhood chestiness' (with or without history of atopic illness)
Smoking history	**15–20+ pack-years**	No or light smoking history
Family history	With or without a history of 'emphysema' 'Chronic bronchitis'	Atopic illness/asthma
Symptoms	**Non-variable** **Shortness of breath on exertion,** cough and sputum with or without wheeze, 'chest tightness'	**Variable** Wheeze, 'chest tightness', cough and sputum in exacerbations
Nocturnal wakening	Rare	**Common**
Morning symptoms	Rapidly relieved by expectoration	Last several hours

The features in **bold** are the particularly relevant ones.

The next step is to evaluate the patient's spirometry. If the spirometry is obstructed and the history is consistent with COPD rather than asthma, the patient's therapy needs to be re-evaluated.

The BTS Guidelines, published in 1997, recommended that oral steroid trials be performed in all patients who had moderate to severe disease – i.e. all those with an FEV_1 less than 50% predicted. However, the Isolde trial demonstrated that inhaled steroids benefit these patients in terms of fewer exacerbations and a reduced rate of decline in health status, and the NICE guidelines recommend their use in patients:

- who have an FEV_1 less than 50% predicted,

- who suffer two or more exacerbations a year, requiring treatment with antibiotics or oral steroids.

It could therefore be argued that formal steroid trials are not needed in these patients, except to exclude a diagnosis of asthma.

In practice, most of the patients from the asthma register who are being re-evaluated to see if they actually have COPD will already be taking inhaled steroids. None of the guidelines offers any advice on how to perform steroid trials on patients who are already, perhaps inappropriately, receiving inhaled steroids.

Where it is suspected that high-dose inhaled steroids are being given inappropriately:

■ Reduce the dose by 25% every three months (as suggested in the BTS *British Guidelines for Asthma Management*).

■ Review the patient frequently, observing for rapidly declining lung function or deterioration of symptoms.

The approach outlined above, whilst not giving rapid results, would seem logical. If a patient with asthma is already optimally controlled on inhaled steroids, any response to an oral steroid trial is likely to be masked, giving a false-negative result. The inhaled steroids may then be discontinued when they are needed. The slow reduction of inhaled steroids is also supported by an observational report from the Isolde trial. When steroids were abruptly withdrawn from patients in the seven-week run-in period to the trial, 32% of the patients suffered an exacerbation.

Reappraisal of the practice asthma register may improve the diagnosis rate in patients with moderate to severe disease and allow more rational prescribing, but it is unlikely to improve the diagnosis rate in patients with mild, largely asymptomatic, disease and those with mild to moderate disease who may be attending with 'chest infections' in the winter. It is an unfortunate fact that, by the time symptoms of COPD become apparent, considerable and irreversible loss of lung function has already occurred. If severe, debilitating, expensive and life-threatening disease is to be prevented, it must be detected early and smoking cessation advice and support given. If awareness of the possibility of COPD is raised with smokers who attend with occasional 'chest infections' and they are screened with spirometry, the detection rate for early COPD is likely to improve.

The role of spirometry in the detection and diagnosis of COPD has already been discussed. However, spirometers are expensive and they must be used properly if the results are not to be meaningless. Incorrectly performed spirometry may result in patients being referred for specialist opinion unnecessarily, or patients needing referral being missed. Training in the correct use and care of equipment and basic interpretation of the results is essential.

A machine that complies with BTS Guidelines for lung function testing and providing the necessary training are likely to cost in excess of £1,000. This may not be practicable for every general practice. Some areas already have open access to spirometry at the local hospital, along similar lines as open access to radiography. The expertise, equipment and facilities for quality control are already available in the hospital, although some extra staffing provision may be needed. Patients, however, may find this less attractive, because it can involve travelling greater distances and thus be less convenient. For a large general practice or a group of smaller practices working co-operatively or a practice with a particular respiratory interest where a machine is likely to be used extensively, the purchase of a spirometer may be a cost-effective option. A third possibility is the provision of mobile community spirometry services. Which of these options is most the practical must be decided at a local level.

The practice nurse's role

Throughout this book we have emphasised the need for a structured approach to diagnosis and management and the need for patient education, involving both the GP and the practice nurse. Their effectiveness with asthma patients has been widely studied but there is a dearth of research relating to COPD. However, it would seem logical that COPD patients will benefit from a similar approach. The fact that COPD and asthma differ has also been emphasised in this book, to stress how important it is that health professionals caring for patients have a sound understanding of those differences and their implications for treatment.

Providing a structured approach to care in COPD requires doctor or nurse time. In practices already running asthma clinics, extending the scope of the clinic to include COPD management – an 'airways clinic' – is one possible approach. Many COPD patients attend 'asthma clinics', so this may be a practicable option.

Appropriately trained nurses have had – and continue to have – a major impact on asthma management. How involved GPs and nurses are in COPD management should depend on their knowledge, interest and expertise. Whatever their role, they must be trained for it and should have been assessed as competent. The

Table 14.2 The role of the practice nurse

Minimum involvement

Maintain a register of known COPD patients

Call COPD patients annually for influenza vaccination

Ensure that COPD patients have received pneumococcal
    vaccination

Encourage patients to stop smoking, and advise them at each visit

Teach and check inhaler technique

Provide information to patients and their relatives about COPD
    – e.g. British Lung Foundation

(The patient is managed and followed up by the GP)

Suggested training:

In-house training

Local study evenings in COPD and smoking cessation

Basic COPD course – e.g. NRTC COPD Short Course

Basic smoking cessation course – e.g. NRTC Smoking Cessation
    Short Course

+ EXPERIENCE

Medium involvement

As for 'Minimum involvement', plus:

Take a basic respiratory history

Carry out diagnostic procedures – e.g. spirometry and reversibility
    testing – when indicated

Update the COPD register

Establish a regular follow-up procedure for COPD patients

Provide basic information and advice on diet and exercise

(The patient is cared for jointly by the GP and the practice nurse)

Training needs:

Spirometry training: caring for the equipment, getting a technically
    acceptable result and basic interpretation – e.g. NRTC
    Spirometry Short Course, ARTP Certificate of Competence

Assessed diploma level training in COPD – e.g. NRTC COPD
    Module

Table 14.2 The role of the practice nurse (*continued*)

+ EXPERIENCE

Maximum involvement

As for 'Medium involvement', plus:

Take a full respiratory history

Perform a basic examination of the patient to assess for hyperinflation, central cyanosis and oedema

Be able to recognise abnormal spirometry

Suggest further investigation – chest x-ray, ECG, full blood count, etc.

Assess disability and handicap

Instigate therapeutic trials and evaluate their effectiveness

Assess the need for pulmonary rehabilitation and refer/instigate as necessary

Advise patients on self-management

Liaise with other appropriate health professionals

Provide regular follow-up and support for patients and their families

(The patient is managed and followed up by the nurse, with GP support and advice)

Training needs:

Spirometry interpretation course

Assessed degree-level training in COPD – e.g. NRTC Advanced COPD Course

© *The National Respiratory Training Centre 1999. Reproduced with permission.*

routine care of asthma patients has, in many practices, been almost completely devolved to nurses. However, COPD patients are usually older, often have multiple pathologies and are generally more difficult to manage. They are a group of patients for whom a team approach is essential. Appropriately trained nurses can develop a great deal of expertise in COPD, but may be relatively inexperienced in the management of, for example, ischaemic heart disease, so it is vital that they recognise their limitations (Table 14.2). Easy communication between members of the team and appreciation of each other's expertise and role are needed.

Protocol and audit

There should be a practice protocol that clearly defines how patients are managed and describes the roles of each member of the primary care team. Patient group directions need to be in place to allow the nurse to carry out reversibility testing (this is a legal requirement). The protocol should be agreed and followed by all members of the team so that the approach is systematic and logical, and patients receive consistent advice. It should follow current guidelines for the care of COPD. Suggestions for what should be considered when formulating a practice protocol are given in Table 14.3.

The effectiveness of your practice's COPD management should be audited, so that standards can be maintained and improved, and any deficiencies highlighted and remedied. Unfortunately, there has been little research to determine which outcome measures should be audited, so the suggestions listed in Table 14.4 are largely based on conjecture, and include General Medical Service contract performance indicators.

For the health professional the proper management of COPD patients can be immensely rewarding and satisfying. Many patients have been dismissed as 'hopeless cases'. They frequently have low self-esteem and poor expectations. Trevor Clay OBE – former Secretary of the Royal College of Nursing (RCN), tireless campaigner for the British Lung Foundation Breathe Easy groups and a COPD sufferer – summed up the problems many COPD patients face when he addressed the RCN Respiratory Nurses Forum:

> 'Our [Breathe Easy's] aim is to remove the phrase 'there's nothing more that can be done' from the vocabulary of health professionals. Not only does it have a devastating effect but it is simply not true. What is meant is that there is no magic, no cure, but there is always something that can be done.'

A greater awareness and understanding of COPD should improve the standard of care that COPD patients receive and should ultimately result in a reduction in the burden that this devastating disease causes.

Table 14.3 Example of a practice protocol

Case finding and maintenance of disease register

- Update diagnosis opportunistically
- Opportunistic and new patient screening
- Systematic search of patient records (aged 40+, recurrent 'chest infection', smoker)
- Reappraisal of practice asthma register

Diagnostic criteria

- Symptoms
- Lung function – preferably spirometry
- Reversibility to bronchodilators and corticosteroids, when indicated
- Other investigations – chest x-ray, ECG, full blood count, etc.

Treatment

- Disease severity recorded
- Response to therapeutic bronchodilator trials measured objectively and recorded
- Stepwise approach to drug treatment and antibiotics

Referral criteria

- Referral for specialist opinion
- Referral for admission during exacerbation
- Referral for pulmonary rehabilitation

Follow-up and recall

- Review and recall of patients on practice register
- Annual review of patients – to include:
  - functional status,
  - BMI,
  - MRC dyspnoea score,
  - response to therapy,
  - exacerbation rate in previous 12 months,
  - FEV_1 in patients with rapidly declining functional status or frequent exacerbation,
  - pulse oximetry if FEV_1 less than 50% predicted,
  - review of management.
- Follow-up of patients admitted to hospital
- Review of patients on long-term oxygen and nebulisers

Table 14.3 Example of a practice protocol (*continued*)

Smoking cessation policy
- Record smoking status and 'tag' patient records
- Discuss and encourage the use of nicotine replacement therapy or bupropion
- Review and recall patients who are 'quitting'

Delegation of care and internal referral policy
- Named GP with overall responsibility
- Role of practice nurse (according to expertise and training)
- Role of support staff

Table 14.4 COPD audit

Audit of process
    Percentage of smokers who have had spirometry performed
    Number of patients on the COPD register
    Number of newly diagnosed patients who have had the diagnosis confirmed by spirometry and reversibility
    Number of patients who were ever diagnosed by spirometry
    Number of patients still smoking
    Number who have had smoking cessation advice
    Number who have had FEV_1 recorded in the previous 27 months
    Number who have had their inhaler technique checked
    Number who have had influenza vaccine in the previous season
    Number vaccinated against pneumococcus

Audit of outcome
    Number of patients still smoking
    Number of emergency admissions
    Number of emergency GP consultations
    Disability scores
    Handicap scores

Further reading

BRITISH THORACIC SOCIETY, ASSOCIATION OF RESPIRATORY TECHNICIANS AND PHYSIOLOGISTS (1994) Guidelines for the measurement of respiratory function. *Respiratory Medicine* **88**: 165–94

BRITISH THORACIC SOCIETY, SCOTTISH INTERCOLLEGIATE GUIDELINES NETWORK (2003) British guideline on the management of asthma. *Thorax* **58** (Suppl 1): i1–i94

NATIONAL INSTITUTE FOR CLINICAL EXCELLENCE (2004) Chronic obstructive pulmonary disease: National clinical guidelines on management of COPD in adults in primary and secondary care. *Thorax* **59** (suppl 1): 1–232

Useful addresses

British Lung Foundation
73–75 Goswell Road
London EC1V 7ER
Tel: 020 7688 5555
Fax: 020 7688 5556
Website: www.lunguk.org

National Respiratory Training Centre
The Athenaeum
10 Church Street
Warwick CV34 4AB
Tel: 01926 493313
Fax: 01926 493224
Website: www.nrtc.org.uk

Glossary

Words shown in *italic* in the definition are also defined in this Glossary

ACE inhibitor angiotensin-converting enzyme inhibitor – a class of drugs used in hypertension and cardiac failure

adaptive aerosol delivery (AAD) an innovative nebuliser system that delivers drug during inhalation only and can be programmed to deliver a precise amount of drug

aerobic exercise exercise to increase the efficiency of the heart and lungs in delivering oxygen to the tissues

air-trapping excess air remaining in the lung at the end of exhalation. This may be due to airway collapse and/or loss of lung elasticity, as in *emphysema*

airway hyper-responsiveness the airways are over-reactive and 'irritable' and more likely to constrict in response to a wide variety of physical and chemical stimuli

alpha-1 antitrypsin (α_1-AT) an *antiprotease* in the blood. Congenital deficiency of alpha-1 antitrypsin is associated with the early presentation (under 40 years of age) of severe *emphysema*

alveolar/capillary interface the surface of the lung where gas exchange occurs

anticholinergic bronchodilator a drug that inhibits the action of acetylcholine on parasympathetic nerve endings in the lungs and dilates airways

antioxidants substances that neutralise oxidants. They occur naturally in foods rich in vitamins C and E, and may help to slow the rate of progression of COPD

antiprotease/elastase enzyme that neutralises protease/elastase (enzymes that destroy lung tissue by digesting *elastin*, one of the proteins that makes up lung parenchyma)

arterial blood gases measurement of the amount of oxygen and carbon dioxide dissolved in the plasma of an arterial blood sample, measured in kilopascals (kPa)

asthma chronic inflammatory condition of the airways, leading to widespread, variable airway obstruction that is reversible spontaneously or with treatment. Long-standing asthma may become unresponsive to treatment

atopy hereditary predisposition to develop allergic *asthma*, rhinitis and eczema. It is associated with high levels of the antibody IgE

beta-2 agonist bronchodilator a drug that stimulates the beta-adrenergic receptors in the lungs, resulting in bronchodilation

Blue Badge (formerly **Orange Badge**) **scheme** a scheme for disabled persons, allowing them to park in restricted areas

'blue bloater' a somewhat outmoded term used to describe a cyanosed COPD patient who is oedematous and at risk of *cor pulmonale*

Borg scale a measure of breathlessness by which the patient quantifies the amount of breathlessness that an activity produces

breath-assisted nebuliser a jet nebuliser that boosts output during inhalation and minimises drug wastage during exhalation

Breathe Easy Club the name of patient support groups facilitated by the British Lung Foundation

bronchiectasis irreversible dilation of the bronchi due to bronchial wall damage, causing chronic cough and mucopurulent sputum

broncho-alveolar lavage a technique used to wash samples of cells from small airways and alveoli. It is performed during bronchoscopy

bronchomotor tone the amount of bronchial muscle contraction (tone) normally present in the airways. This is often increased in COPD patients

bullous emphysema large cyst-like spaces in the lung that compress normal lung tissue. It may be amenable to surgery

chronic bronchitis sputum production that occurs on most days for at least three months in at least two consecutive years (Medical Research Council definition)

chronic obstructive pulmonary disease (COPD) a slowly progressive disorder characterised by airflow obstruction, which does not change markedly over several months (British Thoracic Society definition)

collagen a connective tissue. Deposition of collagen in the basement membrane of small airways contributes to irreversible airflow obstruction

cor pulmonale pulmonary hypertension and right ventricular hypertrophy (and eventual failure) occurring as a result of chronic lung disease. It causes peripheral oedema, raised jugular venous pressure and liver enlargement

corticosteroid reversibility a test done to determine which COPD patients have significant response (an increase in FEV_1 greater than 200ml and 15% of baseline) to steroids and who merit long-term inhaled steroids. Large improvements are indicative of *asthma* rather than COPD. Prednisolone 30mg is given in the morning for two weeks. Alternatively 1000μg per day of beclometasone (or equivalent) is given for six weeks

corticosteroids/steroids hormones produced by the adrenal glands. Synthetic forms are used in COPD for their anti-inflammatory activity, although their long-term use is controversial

cyanosis blueness of the skin due to *hypoxia*. It is a somewhat subjective finding but when *oxygen saturation* falls below 85–90% cyanosis generally becomes apparent

cyclic adenosine monophosphate (cyclic AMP) a substance found in cells that has a crucial role in bronchodilation and reduction of inflammation

cytokines glycoprotein molecules that regulate cell-to-cell communication of the inflammatory response

dynamic airway collapse the tendency of unsupported airways to collapse during forced exhalation

elastase enzyme that digests *elastin*

elastin protein that makes up lung tissue. Its elastic properties contribute to the lung's elastic recoil and helps expel air from the lungs during exhalation

emphysema abnormal permanent enlargement of the air spaces distal to the terminal bronchiole (alveoli) accompanied by destruction of their walls

eosinophil white blood cell. It is characteristically found in the airways of people with *asthma* and is implicated in long-term inflammation and epithelial damage

FEV$_1$ see *forced expired volume*

fibrosing alveolitis a condition resulting in widespread *fibrosis* of the alveoli. It causes progressive breathlessness and a restrictive spirometry pattern

fibrosis scarring and thickening of an organ or tissue by replacement of the original tissue with collagenous fibrous tissue

flow/volume trace a graph produced by a spirometer in which flow rate (in litres per second) is on the vertical axis and volume (in litres) on the horizontal axis

forced expired volume (FEV$_1$) the amount of air that can be exhaled in the first second of a forced blow from maximum inhalation

forced vital capacity (FVC) the total volume of air that can be exhaled from a maximal inhalation to maximal exhalation

gas transfer test (TLco) a test performed in lung function laboratories that determines the ability of the lungs to take up a small amount of carbon monoxide. It is a measure of how efficiently the *alveolar/capillary interface* is working

'guy-rope effect' the support given to small airways by the elastic walls of the alveoli in the lung parenchyma

health status/quality of life a measure of the impact of a disease on a patient's daily life, and social and emotional well-being

Hoover's sign in-drawing of the lower intercostal margins on inhalation

hypercapnia high levels of carbon dioxide in the blood. Levels over 6kPa are generally considered to be abnormal

hypoxia low levels of oxygen in the blood. Levels below 10kPa are generally considered to be abnormal

hypoxic challenge a method of assessing the response of a patient to the reduced oxygen levels they will encounter during air travel

hypoxic respiratory drive a stimulus to breathe that is driven by low levels of oxygen. When patients with this abnormal drive are given high levels of oxygen the stimulus to breathe will be suppressed, resulting in worsening respiratory failure or respiratory arrest

immunoglobulin E (IgE) an antibody. Raised levels of IgE are associated with *atopy* and allergy

inhaled corticosteroids/steroids *corticosteroids* available as beclometasone, budesonide or fluticasone in a variety of inhaler devices

jet nebulisers the most commonly used nebuliser. Atomising the drug solution in the airflow from a compressor or piped gas supply produces the aerosol

leukotriene antagonists a new class of drugs for *asthma* that either block the formation of leukotrienes or block the leukotriene receptors in the lungs

long-term oxygen therapy (LTOT) oxygen given for 15 hours or more a day. It improves life expectancy and may improve health status in chronically hypoxic COPD patients

losartan a recently developed angiotensin II inhibitor that reduces pulmonary artery pressure in COPD

lung volume reduction surgery a new technique developed in the USA to remove 20–30% of the most emphysematous parts of the lung and improve breathlessness

lymphocytes white blood cells involved in the body's immune system

macrophages white blood cells that are involved in phagocytosis and secretion of cytokines that attract and activate neutrophils and other inflammatory cells

mast cells white blood cells that release histamine and other inflammatory mediators. *Immunoglobulin E* is attached to their surfaces

nicotine replacement therapy (NRT) a method of reducing craving and withdrawal symptoms in people attempting to stop smoking. It is available as chewing gum, transdermal patches, inhalator, nasal spray, lozenges and sublingual tablets. It can double success rates

obliterative bronchiolitis widespread fibrotic, inflammatory condition of the small airways. A late and serious complication of lung transplantation, it is frequently fatal in 6–12 months

obstructive sleep apnoea (OSA) upper airway obstruction occurring during sleep. It may result in repeated and significant episodes of hypoxia and severe sleep deprivation. Can cause *cor*

pulmonale and may coexist with COPD. Commonly presents
with daytime somnolence and a history of severe snoring

occupational asthma variable airway obstruction resulting from
exposure to a sensitising agent inhaled at work. Continued
exposure to the causative agent may result in severe, persistent
asthma with irreversibility

osteoporosis demineralisation and atrophy of bone, associated
with an increased risk of fracture. It is most commonly seen in
post-menopausal women but is also associated with long-term
use of oral *corticosteroids*

oxidants see *oxygen radicals/oxidants*

oxygen concentrator electrically powered molecular 'sieve' that
removes nitrogen and carbon dioxide and delivers almost pure
oxygen to the patient. It is a cost-effective method of delivering
long-term oxygen

oxygen cost diagram a measure of disability in which a patient
marks a 10cm line against an activity that induces breathlessness. The disability score is the distance along the line

oxygen radicals/oxidants highly active molecules – found in
tobacco smoke and released by inflammatory cells – that can
damage lung tissue

oxygen saturation the percentage of haemoglobin saturated with
oxygen. It is measured with a pulse oximeter. Normal oxygen
saturation is over 95%. Cyanosis is apparent with a saturation
of between 85% and 90%

peak expiratory flow (PEF) the maximal flow rate that can be
maintained over the first 10 milliseconds of a forced blow

phosphodiesterase inhibitors a group of drugs, including
theophyllines, that increase *cyclic AMP* levels and may reduce
inflammation and cause bronchodilation

photochemical pollutants gases such as ozone, produced by the
action of sunlight on vehicle exhaust gases

'pink puffer' a somewhat outmoded term to describe a COPD
patient who is very breathless but has normal arterial blood gases
and is not at risk of the early development of *cor pulmonale*

pneumococcal vaccination recommended for COPD patients by
the Department of Health although controlled studies of its
effectiveness are lacking

pneumotachograph a device for measuring flow rates. Some electronic spirometers use these to assess flow rates and calculate lung volumes from the flow rates

polycythaemia an abnormal increase in the number of red blood cells. In COPD this can occur as a result of chronic *hypoxia*

pulmonary oedema extravasated fluid in the lung tissue. Commonly caused by left ventricular failure

pulmonary rehabilitation a programme of exercises and education aimed at reducing disability and handicap in chronic respiratory disease.

pulse oximetry a non-invasive method of assessing the amount of haemoglobin that is saturated with oxygen (*oxygen saturation*)

quality of life see *health status*

respiratory drive the stimulus to breathe. The main respiratory centre is in the medulla of the brain

respiratory failure failure to maintain oxygenation. It is usually taken to mean failure to maintain oxygenation above 8kPa

respiratory muscle training breathing exercises aimed at improving respiratory muscle strength and endurance. Its effectiveness in COPD is debatable

restrictive lung disease a disease that causes reduction in lung volumes (FVC and FEV_1) without reduction in flow rates through the airways (FEV_1/FVC ratio normal or high)

sarcoid an inflammatory disease of unknown cause affecting many parts of the body. Chronic sarcoidosis affecting the lungs causes diffuse fibrosis, reduction of lung volumes and, sometimes, airflow obstruction with air-trapping

shuttle walking test a method of assessing walking distance. The patient performs a paced walk between two points 10 metres apart (a shuttle) at an incrementally increasing pace, dictated by 'beeps' on a tape recording, until they are unable to maintain the pace

'silent area' a term used to describe the generation of airways 2–5mm in diameter. Considerable damage can occur in this area without causing symptoms

simple bronchitis chronic mucus production that is not associated with airflow obstruction

small airways disease pathological changes affecting airways 2–5mm in diameter, including occlusion of the airway with mucus, goblet cell hyperplasia, inflammatory changes in the airway wall, fibrosis and smooth muscle hypertrophy

smoking 'pack-years' a method of quantifying cigarette exposure:

$$\frac{\text{Number smoked per day}}{20} \times \text{Number of years smoked}$$

steroids see *corticosteroids*

theophyllines methylxanthine bronchodilator drug with a modest bronchodilator effect in COPD

total lung capacity (TLC) the volume of air in the lungs after maximum inhalation. It comprises the vital capacity and the residual volume

ultrasonic nebulisers nebulisers in which the aerosol is generated by agitating the nebuliser solution with ultrasonic vibrations produced by a piezo crystal

ventilation/perfusion mismatch a situation in which areas of the lung have a blood supply and no air and vice versa. It results in inefficient gas exchange

Venturi mask an oxygen mask that supplies a fixed percentage of oxygen

volume/time trace a graph produced by a spirometer whereby volume is plotted on the vertical axis and time on the horizontal axis

Useful addresses

Association of Respiratory Technology and Physiology
ARTP Administration
Suite 4 Sovereign House
Gate Lane
Boldmere
Birmingham B73 5TT
Tel/Fax: 0845 226 3062
Website: artp.org.uk
Runs training courses on respiratory function testing and assesses/certifies competence in the technique of spirometry

Breathe Easy Club
British Lung Foundation
73–75 Goswell Road
London EC1V 7ER
Tel: 020 7688 5555
Fax: 020 7688 5556
Website: www.lunguk.org
Self-help groups for social contact, support and encouragement

British Lung Foundation
73–75 Goswell Road
London EC1V 7ER
Tel: 020 7688 5555
Fax: 020 7688 5556
Website:
www.britishlungfoundation.com
Association of professionals who fund medical research and provide support and information to people with lung disease. Offers leaflets about suitable gentle exercises and breathing control

British Thoracic Society
17 Doughty Street
London WC1N 2PL
Tel: 020 7831 8778
Fax: 020 7831 8766
Website:
www.brit-thoracic.org.uk
Official body of medical practitioners, nurses, scientists and any professional with an interest in respiratory disease, promoting the interests of patients with lung diseases. For a copy of Spirometry in Practice *see the website:*
www.brit-thoracic.org.uk/pdf/
COPDSpirometryInPractice.pdf
or e-mail copd@imc-group.co.uk
or fax to 01252 845700

Chest, Heart and Stroke Association (Northern Ireland)
21 Dublin Road
Belfast BT2 7HB
Tel: 028 90 320184
Fax: 028 90 333487
Website: www.nichsa.com
For information and advice

Chest, Heart and Stroke (Scotland)
65 North Castle Street
Edinburgh EH2 3LT
Tel: 0131 225 6963
Fax: 0131 220 6313
Website: www.chss.org.uk
For information and advice

General Practice Airways Group (GPIAG)
8th floor, Edgbaston House
3 Duchess Place
Birmingham B16 8NH
Tel: 0121 454 8219
Fax: 01461 207819
Website: www.gpiag.org
Registered charity for healthcare professionals in primary care

Health Development Agency
Holborn Gate
330 High Holborn
London WC1V 7BA
Tel: 020 7430 0850
Fax: 020 7061 3390
Helpline: 0870 121 4194
Website:
www.hda-online.org.uk
Formerly the Health Education Authority; it now deals only with research. Publications on health matters can be ordered via the Helpline

National Respiratory Training Centre
The Athenaeum
10 Church Street
Warwick CV34 4AB
Tel: 01926 493313
Fax: 01926 493224
Website: www.nrtc.org.uk
Courses on respiratory care for all health professionals.
Publications: Simply COPD, Simply Stop Smoking *and others*

Quit (Smoking Quitlines)
England: 0800 00 22 00
Northern Ireland:
028 90 663 281
Scotland: 0800 84 84 84
Wales: 0800 169 0169 (national number)
Website: www.quit.org.uk
For help with trying to stop smoking

**Royal College of Physicians
of Edinburgh**
9 Queen Street
Edinburgh EH2 1JQ
Tel: 0131 225 7324
Fax: 0131 220 3939
Website: www.rcpe.ac.uk/
*Independent professional
organisation promoting the
highest standards in internal
medicine*

*Addresses for breathlessness
questionnaires*

**Chronic Respiratory Disease
Index Questionnaire**
Peggy Austin and
Dr Holger Schünemann
Room 2C12
McMaster University Health
Sciences Centre
Hamilton
Ontario L8N 3Z5
CANADA
Email: austinp@mcmaster.ca
or schuneh@mcmaster.ca

**St George's Respiratory
Questionnaire**
Professor Paul Jones
Division of Physiological
Medicine
St George's Hospital Medical
School
Cranmer Terrace
London SW17 0RE
Email: sadie@sghms.ac.uk

**Breathing Problems
Questionnaire**
Professor Michael Hyland
Department of Psychology
University of Plymouth
Plymouth
Devon PL4 8AA
Email:
mhyland@plymouth.ac.uk

Manufacturers

3M Health Care Ltd
3M House
Morley Street
Loughborough
Leicestershire LE11 1EP
Tel: 01509 611611
Fax: 01509 613105
Website:
www.3mhealthcare.co.uk

Allen & Hanburys Ltd
Stockley Park West
Uxbridge
Middlesex UB11 1BT
Tel: 0800 221 441
Fax: 020 8990 4328
Website: www.gsk.com

AstraZeneca UK Ltd
Horizon Place
600 Capability Green
Luton
Bedfordshire LU1 3LU
Tel: 0800 7830 033
Fax: 01582 838003
Website: astrazeneca.co.uk

Aventis Pharma Ltd
Aventis House
50 Kings Hill Avenue
Kings Hill
West Malling
Kent ME19 4AH
Tel: 01732 584000
Fax: 01732 584080
Website: www.aventis.com

Boehringer Ingelheim Ltd
Ellesfield Avenue
Southern Industrial Estate
Bracknell
Berkshire RG12 8YS
Tel: 01344 424600
Fax: 01344 741444
Website:
www.boehringer-ingelheim.com

Clement Clarke
International Ltd
Unit A
Cartel Business Estate
Edinburgh Way
Harlow
Essex CM20 2TT
Tel: 01279 414969
Fax: 01279 456304
Website:
www.clement-clarke.com

Ferraris Medical Ltd
4 Harforde Court
John Tate Road
Hertford SG13 7NW
Tel: 01992 526300
Fax: 01992 526320
Website:
www.ferrarismedical.com

GlaxoSmithKline
Stockley Park West
Uxbridge
Middlesex UB11 1BT
Tel: 0800 221 441
Fax: 020 8990 4328
Website: www.gsk.com

IVAX Pharmaceuticals
Albert Basin
Armada Way
Royal Docks
London E16 2QJ
Tel: 08705 020304
Fax: 08705 323334
Website: www.ivax.co.uk

Micro Medical
Quayside
Chatham Maritime
Chatham
Kent ME4 4QY
Tel: 01634 893500
Fax: 01634 893600
Website:
www.micromedical.co.uk

Napp Pharmaceuticals
Cambridge Science Park
Milton Road
Cambridge CB4 0GW
Tel: 01223 424444
Fax: 01223 424441
Website: www.napp.co.uk

Profile Respiratory Systems
Heath Place
Bognor Regis
West Sussex PO22 9SL
Tel: 01243 840888
Fax: 01243 846100
Website: www.profilehs.com

Vitalograph Ltd
Maids Moreton
Buckingham MK18 1SW
Tel: 01280 827110
Fax: 01280 823302
Website: www.vitalograph.co.uk

Website

www.goldcopd.com
Recommends effective COPD management and prevention strategies for use in all countries. Gives the names and contact details of various national and international members of the group

Index

NOTE: page numbers in *italic* refer to figures or tables; '*g*' after a page number indicates an entry in the Glossary.

ACE (angiotensin-converting enzyme) inhibitors 156, 184, 197*g*

N-acetyl cysteine 178, 183

activity curtailment 5, 29, 59–62, *114*
  loss of muscle mass 138–9
  occupational therapy 117
  social and psychological issues 139–41
  see also assessment; breathlessness; exercise

acute exacerbations of COPD 23
  antibiotics 147, 150–1, 154
  associated conditions 156
  bronchodilators 145
  corticosteroid therapy 99–100
  definition 146, 167
  follow-up 152
  GOLD guidelines 179
  home/hospital choice 145, *149*, 155
  infective 145
  main points 145–6
  management 148, 167
  natural history 148–50
  NICE guidelines 167
  prevention 152–3
  quality of life 150, 163
  recurrent 152, 163

respiratory failure 155–6
  self-management 145, 153–4
  specialist referral 156, *157*
  studies 146, 147, 148, 150, 152, 154
  symptoms 147, 167
  treatment 84, 87, 88, 150–2, 167
  triggers 147–8

admission to hospital *see* hospital admission

advice 116–18, 120
  see also information

age
  adolescents and smoking 69
  elderly people
    bronchodilators 84–5
    corticosteroid therapy 100
    pneumococcal infections 137
    theophylline 88
  increase as risk factor 13–14
  lung function 12, *13*
  lung transplants 126, 136
  presentation of symptoms 13
  specialist referral *157*

AHR (airway hyper-responsiveness) 15, 197*g*

air pollution 16, 147

air-trapping in lungs 29, 54, 197*g*

airflow obstruction 3, 10, 35
  acute exacerbations 145, 147
  conditions likely to cause obstructive/restrictive disease *41*
  gradations (mild, moderate, severe) 163–4, *164*

Have you found **Chronic Obstructive Pulmonary Disease in Primary Care** useful and practical? If so, you may be interested in these other titles from Class Publishing.

The 'at your fingertips' series

'Woe betide any clinicians or nurses whose patients have read this invaluable source of down-to-earth information when they have not.' – The Lancet

Our best-selling series, the *'at your fingertips'* guides seek to help those who, having been diagnosed with a condition, have countless questions that need answering. These essential handbooks answer all the questions that patients want to know about their health and condition. The formula for the series follows a question-and-answer format, with real questions from sufferers and their families answered by medical experts at the top of their fields, without the jargon of medical texts. All these books are packed full of practical information for patients and their families.

Each title is only £14.99 plus p&p. Topics covered range from diagnosis to treatment, and from relationships to welfare entitlements.

'Contains the answers the doctor wishes he had given if only he'd had the time.' – DR THOMAS STUTTAFORD, *The Times*

Titles currently available (or coming soon*):

Acne • Allergies • Asthma • Beating Depression • Cancer
COPD • Dementia – Alzheimer's & other dementias • Diabetes*
Epilepsy • Gout • Heart Health • High Blood Pressure
Kidney Dialysis & Transplants • Motor Neurone Disease
Multiple Sclerosis • Osteoporosis • Parkinson's • Psoriasis
Sexual Health for Men • Stroke

COPD – the 'at your fingertips' guide $\qquad$ £14.99
Dr Jon Miles and June Roberts

- Provides comprehensive and up-to-date information from leading medical experts

- Cuts out confusing medical jargon and explains facts in plain English

- Tackles the questions that patients may feel uneasy asking doctors

- Contains details of national organisations offering further help and support

- Medically accurate information on a whole range of topics from diagnosis and treatment, to management and self-help and much much more

In this invaluable reference guide two leading experts answer hundreds of patients' questions. This practical manual is packed full of sensible advice that is easy to act upon, and gives comprehensive, medically accurate information on COPD and other forms of respiratory problems in an easy-to-understand format.

COPD – the 'at your fingertips' guide outlines the different care options that are available and suggests a variety of strategies for coping as well as telling you where to go for help and guidance. The expert authors also address the physical and emotional upheaval that COPD can bring. They discuss its impact on the whole family, offering positive help and advice.

Due for publication Summer 2004

Asthma – the 'at your fingertips' guide

NEW! Third Edition   £14.99

Dr Mark Levy, Professor Sean Hilton and Greta Barnes MBE

'Having asthma should not stop you leading a full and active life. With full knowledge of my condition, the correct treatment and a desire to succeed, I became an Olympic champion. This book gives you the knowledge. Don't limit yourself.'

ADRIAN MOOREHOUSE MBE, Olympic Gold Medallist

Asthma – the 'at your fingertips' guide gives patients – and their families – clear and positive answers to all the questions that they will want to ask about asthma. It is packed full of practical advice and useful tips. The book is written in a straightforward way, with a comprehensive index so that readers can find the information they need quickly.

For anyone in who has asthma – or asthma in the family – this book will be an invaluable source of reference. It gives the confidence needed to deal with asthma successfully, by answering all your questions about it, such as:

- What are the warning signs of an asthma attack?

- How can I find the best inhaler device for me?

- Why is my asthma worse at night?

- I am expecting my first child: will I get breathing difficulties in labour?

- What precautions should we take for our child on holiday?

- Will my son grow out of his asthma or will it get worse?

This book also:

- Includes up-to-date information on new treatments and self-management plans;

- Contains everything parents need to know to deal with their child's asthma with confidence;

- PLUS! A 20-page colour guide to the latest asthma equipment and how to use it.

Demonstrates the most effective ways of managing asthma. Once patients understand how to control their condition, they are more likely to enjoy a full and active life!

Allergies – the 'at your fingertips' guide £14.99
Dr Joanne Clough

'An excellent book which deserves to be on the bookshelf of every family.'
DR CSABA RUSZNAK, Medical Director, British Allergy Foundation

Allergies – the 'at your fingertips' guide provides concise, practical information about allergies: what they are, how they develop and what to do about them. Written in straightforward, non-medical language, this essential guide gives patients 100% medically accurate information on allergies in an easy-to-understand format.

Allergies – the 'at your fingertips' guide contains chapters on:

Asthma and allergy • Allergies and the skin • Hayfever and rhinitis
Food and bowel allergies • Life threatening allergies
Diagnosing your allergies • Allergies at work

This unique reference guide:

- Answers 312 real questions from people with allergies;
- Is 100% accurate and up-to-date answers from a leading medical expert;
- Offers practical advice on how to manage allergies in day-to-day life;
- Contains everything parents need to know to deal with their child's allergy with confidence;
- Is jargon-free, with all medical terminology explained in straightforward language;
- Tells you exactly what to do in an emergency;
- Answers the questions you may feel uneasy asking your doctor.

At last – sensible, practical advice on allergies from an experienced medical expert.

Providing Diabetes Care in General Practice

Fourth Edition   £24.99

Mary MacKinnon

'It is a real contribution to a modern understanding of so many aspects of diabetes.'
PROFESSOR HARRY KEEN, Former Vice President of Diabetes UK

Mary MacKinnon's 'bible' gives you all the back-up and information you need to run a high-quality, effective diabetes service within your practice. Armed with this reference manual, your team will be able to provide high standards of patient care at realistic cost. This tried-and-tested system defines roles for each member of the primary care team from the GP to the receptionist, and anticipates problems before they arise, ensuring top-quality care without any increase in cost to you.

- How to guarantee top-quality care

- What equipment and resources you need

- How to organise recall and follow-up effectively

- All the education your patients – and you – will need to know

Chapters include:

Diabetes – an overview • The St Vincent Declaration Responsibilities of those involved in the provision of diabetes care Educational needs of the team • Diabetes mellitus in the UK The symptoms of diabetes mellitus • Providing the service Control of blood glucose levels • Eye care and screening Foot care and surveillance • Monitoring and audit of practice diabetes care • History of the condition • Type 1 diabetes Type 2 diabetes • Other categories of diabetes • Other causes of diabetes • The complications of diabetes • Conclusion

'The complete guide for the primary health care team.'
DR MICHAEL HALL, Chairman of Diabetes UK

Vital Diabetes – Second Edition   £14.99

Dr Charles Fox and Mary MacKinnon

'Full of the kind of essential and up-to-date information you need to deliver the best practice in diabetes care.'

M. CARPENTER, *Diabetes Grapevine*

Vital Diabetes gives you:

- Clear and concise information at a glance;

- The confidence to know that your patients are getting the best advice on treatment and self-care;

- Patient (and carer) information you can photocopy for patients to take away with them, whenever they need it;

- All the vital facts and figures about diabetes, for your information and use.

If you are involved in managing diabetes in your practice, it is a superhuman task, especially with treatment guidelines changing all the time in light of new evidence. *Vital Diabetes* is here to help. Written by two experts in the field, Dr Charles Fox and Mary MacKinnon, this book will give you all the back-up you need for best practice in diabetes care, enabling you to keep up with the fast-changing world of diabetes.

Subjects covered include:

Impact and new insights • Screening and identification • How to manage type 2 diabetes • How to control blood glucose levels How to reduce long-term complications of diabetes • How to manage type 1 diabetes • How to manage pregnancy and gestational diabetes • Living with diabetes • Emergencies and illness • Monitoring care in the practice • Glossary of terms Resources • Training/continuing education

Vital facts and figures for anyone involved in diabetes care – in just 96 pages!!

PRIORITY ORDER FORM

Cut out or photocopy this form and send it (post free in the UK) to:

Class Publishing Priority Service, FREEPOST, London W6 7BR

Please send me urgently (*tick below*)

*No. of
copies*

*Post included
price per copy
(UK only)*

☐ Chronic Obstructive Pulmonary Disease in Primary Care   £32.99
(ISBN 1 85959 104 3)

☐ COPD – the 'at your fingertips' guide (ISBN 1 85959 045 4)   £17.99

☐ Asthma – the 'at your fingertips' guide (ISBN 1 85959 006 3)   £17.99

☐ Allergies – the 'at your fingertips' guide (ISBN 1 872362 52 4)   £17.99

☐ Providing Diabetes Care in General Practice   £27.99
(ISBN 1 85959 048 9)

☐ Vital Diabetes (ISBN 1 872362 93 1)   £17.99

Total _____

EASY WAYS TO PAY

Cheque: I enclose a cheque payable to Class Publishing for   _____

Credit card: Please debit my Mastercard ☐ Visa ☐ Amex ☐ Switch ☐

Card no. _____   Expiry date _____

Name _____

My address for delivery is _____

Town _____

County _____   Postcode _____

Telephone number (*in case of query*) _____

Credit card billing address (*if different from above*) _____

Town _____

County _____   Postcode _____

*Class Publishing's guarantee: remember that if, for any reason, you are not satisfied
with these books, we will refund all your money, without any questions asked.
Prices and VAT rates may be altered for reasons beyond our control.*